Heroin Addiction and the British System, Volume I
Origins and Evolution

The 'British System' of dealing with opiate addiction has, for half a century, been notable for its flexibility and its capacity to adapt to changing circumstances. Because of this it has attracted considerable international interest, although it is rarely fully understood or accurately represented.

Presenting a comprehensive account of the development of policies and treatments, *Heroin Addiction and the British System* brings together the perspectives of policy-makers, practitioners, researchers and social commentators. These two volumes contribute to a proper understanding of how policy and practice have evolved so that lessons for future policy and practice may be identified.

Volume I of *Heroin Addiction and the British System* deals with the 'Origins and Evolution' of the drugs problem in the UK, examining the personal, social and political phenomena from historical and contemporary perspectives. It is a unique source of reference for students, researchers, healthcare professionals and drug agencies both in the UK and overseas.

Professor John Strang is Director of the National Addiction Centre at the Institute of Psychiatry, King's College London and is Clinical Director of the Addictions Treatment Services for South London and the Maudsley. **Professor Michael Gossop** is a leading researcher at the National Addiction Centre at the Institute of Psychiatry, King's College London and Head of Research, Addictions, at the Maudsley Hospital.

Heroin Addiction and the British System, Volume I

Origins and Evolution

Edited by John Strang and Michael Gossop

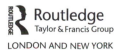
Routledge
Taylor & Francis Group

LONDON AND NEW YORK

First published 2005
by Routledge
2 Park Square, Milton Park, Abingdon, Oxon, OX14 4RN

Simultaneously published in the USA and Canada
by Routledge
270 Madison Ave, New York, NY 10016

Routledge is an imprint of the Taylor & Francis Group

Typeset in Times NR by Graphicraft Limited, Hong Kong
Printed and bound in Great Britain by MPG Books Ltd,
Bodmin, Cornwall

British Library Cataloguing in Publication Data
A catalogue record for this book is available from the British Library

Library of Congress Cataloging in Publication Data
A catalog record has been requested

ISBN 0–415–29814–8 (hbk)
ISBN 0–415–29815–6 (pbk)

Contents

Illustrations

Figures

Tables

Contributors

The editors

John Strang Professor John Strang is Director of the National Addiction Centre (Institute of Psychiatry, King's College London), where he leads the multi-disciplinary treatment and policy research activities and also a Masters degree in the Addictions within the University of London. He is also Clinical Director of the Drug, Alcohol and Smoking Cessation Services of the South London and Maudsley NHS Trust. He was the special consultant advisor on drug treatment services to the Department of Health (England) from 1986 to 2003.

Michael Gossop Professor Michael Gossop is a leading researcher at the National Addiction Centre (Institute of Psychiatry, King's College London), and heads the addictions treatment research at the Maudsley and Bethlem Royal Hospitals. In the mid-1990s, he was responsible for devising and initiating the influential NTORS (National Treatment Outcome Research Study) studying long-term outcome from selected key modalities of treatment in the addictions field.

Chapter authors – Volume I

Virginia Berridge Professor Virginia Berridge is Professor of History at the London School of Hygiene and Tropical Medicine and Head of the History Centre. Her work as a historian has always included a special interest in opiate use in Britain from the Victorian era onwards, as well as changing perceptions of drug and alcohol problems and related public health challenges, notably the development of HIV/AIDS policy.

Thomas Bewley Dr Thomas Bewley was a key figure in the establishment of the drug clinics during the 1960s and worked for many years as a consultant psychiatrist in the substance misuse services at St Thomas's Hospital in the centre of London. He is also a past President of the Royal College of Psychiatrists.

Angela Burr Dr Angela Burr conducted some of the earliest work in the UK into the new patterns of drug use amongst disaffected youth in the 1970s and 1980s. As an anthropologist, she contributed a distinct perspective to understanding of these changes, and she became actively involved in the work of local action responses.

Mark Gilman Mark Gilman is North East Regional Manager of the National Treatment Agency for Substance Misuse in England. Prior to this, he was a research worker, before moving to work, for the next 15 years, with the Lifeline Project in Manchester with whom he was actively involved in new harm-reduction developments.

Paul Griffiths Paul Griffiths is a sociologist who worked at the National Addiction Centre in London during the 1980s and 1990s, where he co-ordinated new research projects into routes of drug administration, and particularly into the spread of chasing the dragon. He has also worked for UNDCP in Vienna, and is currently Head of Epidemiology for the EMCDDA in Lisbon.

Rachel Lart Rachel Lart is a Lecturer in Social Policy at the School for Policy Studies, University of Bristol. She was involved with evaluation of syringe exchanges during the 1990s. More recent research work has been on broader issues in social policy, and she is currently involved in an evaluation of supported housing for drug and alcohol users.

Roger Lewis Roger Lewis worked at Release (a campaigning and legal advice service for drug users) during the 1970s; he also worked on the Drug Indicators Project in north London during the 1980s. One of his main research interests was drug markets and drug trafficking. (Roger Lewis died in 2000 at the age of 56 years.)

Peter McDermott Peter McDermott has extensive experience of drug education projects. He has worked on a range of research projects for the Mersey Drug Training and Information Centre, including monitoring needle exchange use; action research projects on drug use and risk behaviour among prostitutes; and risk behaviours by injecting drug users not in contact with treatment services. He has long-standing interests in service user involvement and patient advocacy.

Howard Parker Professor Howard Parker is Emeritus Professor in the Department of Applied Social Science at Manchester University. During the 1980s he conducted a major study into the emergent heroin problem in Merseyside, and has since continued to look at new patterns of drug use amongst young people in England and Wales.

Diana Patterson Dr Diana Patterson works as a consultant psychiatrist in Addictions, in Belfast, and is also Honorary Senior Lecturer at the Queen's

University, Belfast. From 1991 to 2001 she chaired the Northern Ireland Committee on Drug Misuse. She currently chairs the Treatment Working Group of the Drug and Alcohol Strategy for Northern Ireland.

Geoffrey Pearson Professor Geoffrey Pearson is Professor of Criminology at Goldsmiths College, University of London, and Editor of the *British Journal of Criminology*. During the 1980s he led a research study exploring the regional diversity of patterns of heroin use among young people in the north of England.

N. H. (Raj) Rathod Dr Raj Rathod is a consultant psychiatrist. During the 1960s, at a time when heroin problems were beginning to spread outwards from central London, he was instrumental in setting up a drug dependence clinic in Crawley, a new town just outside Greater London experiencing a heroin epidemic, and was actively involved in conducting research into these young heroin users and their networks.

Roy Robertson Dr James Roy Robertson is a general practitioner at the Muirhouse Medical Group in Edinburgh. He was a key figure in identifying the outbreak of HIV infection among drug injectors in Edinburgh during the 1980s and has continued to play an important role in the research into injecting drug problems in Scotland and the development of primary care services for drug misusers.

Bing Spear Bing Spear worked in the Home Office Drugs Branch from 1952–1986 and was its Chief Inspector from 1977. He had a detailed knowledge and understanding of drug addicts and their problems, and his views were influential among all who worked in the drugs field at that time. (Bing Spear died in 1995 at the age of 67 years.)

Gerry Stimson Professor Gerry Stimson is a medical sociologist who has worked in the drugs field since the late 1960s. He has had an active interest in changes in drugs policy, including the study of needle exchange schemes and harm reduction practices and policies. He is now Director of the Centre for Research on Drugs and Health Behaviour and Head, Department of Social Science and Medicine, Imperial College London.

David Turner David Turner was Director of the Standing Conference on Drug Abuse from 1977–1994, with extensive experience of the workings of the voluntary sector drug services. He was a member of the ACMD from 1978 to 1994, and is currently an adviser to the Italian National Observatory on Drugs and Drug Addiction and Project Co-ordinator for CeIS (Italian Centre for Solidarity) in Rome.

Tom Waller Dr Tom Waller was a general practitioner who had a longstanding special interest in the treatment of drug misusers in primary care settings. He worked in a variety of settings, including City Roads crisis intervention centre in London. He was an active campaigner about the importance of hepatitis C and the need for improved prevention and treatment. (Tom Waller died in 2003 at the age of 59 years.)

Chapter 1

Misreported and misunderstood

The 'British System' of drug policy

John Strang and Michael Gossop (the Editors)

One minute you can see it clearly; the next minute it seems to have vanished, and you realise that you're just not looking in the right place. Like trying to make out the features of a landscape, it seems easier to see the overall shape from far away. The coastal escarpment, the city smog, an evening mist – these are all obvious when observed from afar, and yet go almost unnoticed by the observer on the spot. And so it is with the British System.

The British System is not set down in law, it is not described on tablets of stone. Its imprint at a particular point in time may be discernible within some legislation, but it is not defined by that legislation. Nor is it constant over time, or even geography. Get a clear sighting today, and tomorrow it may already be different. However, it is this absence of any pre-ordained form or structure which perhaps confers on the 'British System' its most impressive feature – its capacity to adapt to the changed circumstances of the day.

Initially, it is tempting to conclude that, on the basis of the differences that may be seen from one decade to the next, there is no British System. Or that, if there ever was a British System, it is now dead. However, to reach this conclusion would be to overlook the very feature which is the quintessential characteristic of the British System – its lack of rigid form and hence its potentially greater capacity to be intuitively reactive to changed circumstances.

The origins of these two volumes

The British System is confusing for many of us. We are often uncertain what is being meant by the phrase when asked to comment upon it, and hence we are torn this way and that about whether we are trying to defend or attack some particular characteristic. Indeed, we are often uncertain about whether we welcome its existence or resent its lack of direction.

The British System has shown itself in diverse ways at different points in time, and has significantly influenced the British response to a variety of stages of the 'drugs problem' at different points in history. These instances of the British System are sometimes handed down as folklore or oral history:

however such transfer of information between the generations is itself a living process so that the later accounts are themselves adapted to the circumstances of the intervening period.

We have been keen to gather, within this book, first-hand accounts of different stages of the British System. And so the chapters in these two volumes are, in many instances, first-hand accounts from key informants who were often themselves an active part of the phenomena described in the particular chapter. The original role played by these contributors will vary – for some they may have been government officials, or senior clinicians, or perhaps drug users seeking (or rejecting) some particular offered treatment. But for all of them, we have asked that they seek out the accurate historical facts and provide as objective a commentary as possible, making maximum use of the distance in time that now exists to increase their capacity for reflection and objective scrutiny. For many of the contributors, this has been a challenging task, with the need to re-examine old data and old values, and we are particularly grateful to them – we believe that the effort in construction of these chapters and the resulting special contribution are evident on reading the individual accounts.

These two volumes also draw on a selection of the material which we, as editors, brought together in an earlier smaller volume *Heroin Addiction and Drug Policy: The British System* which was published in hardback form in 1994. A small number of the chapters from this earlier single volume have been brought forward into the current two-volume edition, especially when we have judged that the individual chapter was particularly important to a proper understanding of the British System as a whole. This has included the reproduction of chapters from authors who have sadly died in the intervening years – former friends and colleagues including Philip Connell, Roger Lewis and Bing Spear. Additionally we have to record, with great sadness, the recent death of the contributor of one of the new chapters – Tom Waller.

Who is the book for?

In the past, the widespread misunderstanding and misrepresentations of the British System could perhaps have been partly excused by the limited opportunity to be properly familiar with its true features. Now, in this linked pair of books, the reader is invited on two illustrated journeys. In the first volume, *Origins and Evolution*, the focus is on achieving a proper understanding of some of the significant developments and the evolution of the drugs problem in the UK, so as to understand the nature of the problem to which the British System was expected to be a response (a quick overview of this first volume is presented in the next few pages). In the second volume, *Treatment and Policy Responses*, the different forms of treatment response which have been employed over the last century are individually explored, either as initiatives which would have been identifiable at the time as new initiatives, or alternatively as broad themes within the British System which can be seen more clearly over the longer time frame (an overview of this second volume is presented at the beginning of this second book).

There is considerable international fascination with the British System, and this fascination itself warrants careful consideration. Certainly the fascination has existed for many decades, and appears to become greater as the distance from the UK increases. At its best, this international interest is a healthy expression of scientific inquiry and dialogue within the global invisible college, between scientists searching truth and objectivity in their examination of different drug policies around the world. Such enquiry and dialogue with colleagues internationally is stimulating, thought-provoking and is a privilege. At its worst, the international interest is little more than the plundering of different cultures and circumstances, searching only for items which reinforce beliefs and positions already rigidly held, and with consideration of the observations only for their relevance in the homeland. Such blinkered inquiry must be identified early, so that limits can be placed on the time and energy that are expended fruitlessly trying to convey the diversity and richness of the true British System.

Overview of Volume I – understanding the problems confronting the British System

An early defining point of the British System was the Rolleston Report of 1926, following which the UK pursued a medically-orientated response to the very small existing problem of opiate addiction, and thereby followed a very different path from the increasingly control-orientated approach being pursued in the US. So much is attributed to the Rolleston Report, and yet there is often little awareness and understanding of its origins, its objectives and its impact. The chapter from Virginia Berridge gives the reader a real understanding of the true significance and contribution of this seminal report.

Up until the 1960s, the UK had a very different type of opiate addiction problem from the typical problem of today. For example the opiate addict was more likely to be female, middle-aged or elderly, and from the middle classes; a substantial minority were themselves doctors or allied professionals. In this quiet stable situation, occasional ripples would occur – and ultimately the tidal wave of the drugs explosion of the 1960s. In a chapter brought forward from the smaller single-volume 1994 book on the British System, we have reproduced the classic description from the late Bing Spear of the early years of opiate addiction in the UK.

The old explanations were no longer adequate for describing or understanding the drugs explosion of the 1960s. For the first time, heroin was being selectively sought, was being injected intravenously by adolescents and young adults, and was being taken in an explicitly hedonistic and social context. This was a new type of problem, and a new analysis was required in order to prepare a more suitable response. In a new chapter describing this important reappraisal in the 1960s, Thomas Bewley re-captures the sense of urgency which created the combined public and professional commitment to the establishment of a newer, better, British System.

Heroin was hitting communities who had never been hit before. Heroin was no longer restricted to London or other major cities. Towns were touched by heroin addiction for the first time, and this socially infectious condition could be tracked as it spread like an infectious disease. One of the classic descriptions of the time was that of the arrival and spread of heroin addiction through Crawley New Town. Raj Rathod revisits this important early epidemiological study, and also brings matters up to date with an account of the subsequent developments for the individuals and the Crawley community.

As if the heroin problem wasn't enough to contend with in the early 1970s, intravenous barbiturate abuse was then added to the cocktail, especially in the London area. The system was stretched to, and often beyond, its limits. Intravenous barbiturates abuse was not only associated with its own distinctive physical complications, but also brought a particularly high risk of overdose deaths. Indeed, this intravenous barbiturate problem was the birthright of City Roads. Angela Burr leads us through a description of this traumatic period and the responses to this new manifestation of youthful drug abuse.

A new type of heroin user was seen for the first time during the 1980s. Whilst the drug use of the 1960s had often been associated with a deliberately anti-establishment stance, the new heroin use of the 1980s seemed to be more directly related to socio-economic disadvantage, to the lack of alternative identity, and, gradually, to a position where such drug use was just part of the new circumstances of the day. Howard Parker guides us through these important observations, and incorporates appropriate material from his classic studies at the time and subsequently, which have shown themselves to be applicable to the wider drug-using youth groups across the UK.

The caricature of the drug dealer may satisfy the needs of the tabloid journalist and reader, but it woefully fails to capture the complexity and the interactive nature of the trading and distribution mechanisms for illicit heroin in the UK (and elsewhere). We have consequently included a chapter by the late Roger Lewis, which gives an excellent insight into this area, and which was previously published in the earlier smaller British System book.

The local diversity of the drug problem is extraordinary. Why should one town be radically different from another, apparently similar, town 20 miles away? But differences there are, and major ones at that – with major differences not only in the size of the problem but also in the very drugs being used, the routes by which they are used, and the social contexts within which the drug use was occurring. Geoff Pearson and Mark Gilman guide us through this intriguing territory to gain a better understanding of the reasons behind these startling local and regional variations.

AIDS has had a profound effect on drug policy everywhere, and it now seems obvious that it should have prompted a major review of British drug policy. However, in the mid-1980s when Edinburgh GP Roy Robertson stumbled across the UK's first explosive outbreak amongst injecting drug misusers, it was far from clear what the implications would be – on those responsible for determining drug policy, as well as on drug misusers themselves.

Mersey became, in the second half of the 1980s, a cauldron of creativity and chaos. In a manner which is hard even to contemplate in most other countries and localities, 'thinking the unthinkable' became commonplace. The challenge then became to find a mechanism for determining which unthinkable thoughts were genuine flashes of inspiration, and which were best left unthought. Radical rethinking, politics, and conflicts between egos – all formed part of the chemistry in the cauldron. As a key player on the inside, Peter McDermott saw, breathed and lived many of the key events, and now provides us with a very special retrospective account of this extraordinary period.

Heroin isn't just heroin any more. Brown or white? South-West Asian or South-East Asian? Base or salt? For chasing or injecting? These features matter greatly, and have a direct influence on whether their heroin is taken by injection or by 'chasing the dragon'. And yet policy makers and practitioners continue to behave as if all heroin is the same. John Strang, Paul Griffiths and Michael Gossop give an overview of the significance of the different types of heroin, their positions in the UK market, and the possible overlooked opportunities for more constructive ways of influencing the heroin trade.

Northern Ireland has historically been most famous for its civil strife and sectarian battles. Strangely, and counter-intuitively, it is a part of the UK with a surprisingly small opiate addiction problem. Problems do exist, but there is a much lower per capita rate of opiate addiction problems in Northern Ireland compared with virtually any other parts of the UK with comparable population density. Diana Patterson has been actively involved strategically as well as clinically, and gives us an excellent insight into this interesting situation.

Is drug policy determined at the local level or at the national level? In a chapter which we have reproduced from the earlier British System book, Gerry Stimson and Rachel Lart explore the changing relationship between the state and local practice with regard to drug policy through the twentieth century, and chart how this relationship has changed over time with the eventual development of explicit public national drugs strategy documents by the end of the century.

Non-governmental organisations, or the 'voluntary sector' or 'non-statutory sector' as they are more usually called in the UK, have always been an important part of drugs service provision in the UK and have been particularly important for introducing missing components of care in the early stages of their introduction to the UK. However, from the 1980s onwards, the size, number, level of funding, and extent of influence of these voluntary sector organisations has grown extraordinarily, so that in many ways they have now become the new 'establishment'. David Turner prepared an important insightful overview of these developments and their significance for the voluntary sector, which was published in the earlier British System book, and which is reproduced here.

The arrival of HIV and AIDS awareness prompted much more than just an adaptation of services to address this new health threat. It prompted a fundamental reconsideration of the objectives and methods of British drugs strategy. The result was a strengthened legitimacy to the approach of harm reduction (even though this phrase was not used extensively until the late 1980s). However, amid the congratulations, it is also necessary to look at areas where the fine rhetoric has still not yet been converted into reality, or where the policy has failed to be protective (for example, against hepatitis C), and also to look for harm reduction opportunities which are not yet being properly explored. John Strang was actively involved in the HIV-driven policy reviews of UK drug policy in the late 1980s and 1990s, and guides the reader through a measured examination, 15 years on, of what can be seen to have occurred.

Hepatitis C has been described as the sleeping giant, and there can be no doubt that, as it wakes, its impact will be catastrophic to injecting drug misusers over the coming decades. So why is the British System sleeping also? The passivity of the response to hepatitis C is in stark contrast to the urgency of the response to HIV in the 1980s. Why? The late Tom Waller guides us through the recent developments, the key issues, and the relevant initiatives (or absence of these initiatives), and sounds an urgent wake-up call for the sleeping British System.

Chapter 2

The 'British System' and its history

Myth and reality

Virginia Berridge

(This chapter draws substantially from the book *Opium and the People. Opiate Use and Drug Control Policy in Nineteenth and Early Twentieth Century England* (expanded edition), London, Free Association Books, 1999, by Virginia Berridge.)

Three 'British Systems'

The 'British System' is a term used to categorise the form of drug control policy established in Britain in the 1920s by the 1926 Rolleston Report. In general, it is taken to mean a medically based system of prescribing opiates to addicts, often on a long-term basis. Its symbolic importance has been considerable. This chapter concentrates on that Report, but there have in fact been at least three 'British Systems' in place from the eighteenth and nineteenth centuries. There was the lay/commercial system of control, which operated until the middle of the nineteenth century; the system of pharmaceutical regulation established in 1868; and the medico-penal system, which received its final legitimisation through Rolleston. Different British Systems have operated at different times and in different relationships to each other. The story of Rolleston and its impact demonstrates how a particular medico-legal form of control came to predominate.

The 'British System' before Rolleston: lay/commercial and pharmaceutical models of control

Drug control in the eighteenth and first half of the nineteenth centuries was based on a mixed commercial and lay system. Opium was freely imported, primarily from Turkey, with commercial distribution in London through opium brokers. Once imported, it passed through a mechanism of wholesaling and retailing which finally brought it within reach of the ordinary consumer of the drug. The opium stocks of the wholesalers were available to any dealer who chose to purchase. Pharmacists and apothecaries, grocers and general dealers all sent in their orders. The carriers' carts would bring out fifty-six-pound lots of raw opium or gallons of laudanum for delivery; or opium arrived regularly by parcel post. Laudanum and other opiate-based preparations were to be found in a range of shops from high street pharmacies to back street corner shops crowded with food, clothing, materials and other drugs. In the small corner shops, 'They put down their penny and get opium', and opium was part of the fabric of a culture where self-medication was the norm and access to formal medical care extremely limited. Opium was a commodity like any other. But, like some other commodities within a largely unregulated system, open sale did present problems. Quality could be variable and adulteration became more marked with the change to an urban society. Poppyhead tea brewed at home was replaced by commercially produced laudanum or other opium products like Godfrey's or paregoric, bought from the local druggist or grocer. Accidental overdosing was quite common.

These and other issues were what lay behind the transition to the second British System in the middle of the nineteenth century. This was the system of pharmaceutical regulation. Of course there were also other issues at stake. One – and a continuing theme in drug policy – was the question of professional status. Pharmacists were establishing a profession of pharmaceutical chemists at this time, based on the existing chemists and druggists and apothecaries, whose main concern was dispensing. Specialist status meant preventing unqualified people from selling drugs, and trying also to regulate the ways in which the general public controlled their own medication. Opium, as such a widely used commodity, naturally came into the story. The 1868 Pharmacy Act subjected opium to pharmaceutical control, but with minimal restrictions (after representations from pharmacists in the Fens, an area of particularly high sale, who did not want their trade destroyed). The Act specifically excluded patent medicines, many of which were opium based.

Further controls over patent medicines were put in place in the 1890s. So the century ended not with one system replacing another, but rather with overlapping systems. There was still a lay/commercial system; and a pharmaceutical one as well, also with a strong commercial element. We next need to consider why and how these systems gave place in the early twentieth century to different forms of control. Why the change? The answer must be sought in a complex of issues, both domestic and international; within Britain, declining cultural acceptability of the drugs and changed positioning of the medical profession, including the impact of new technology; outside Britain, opium's role as an international commodity and the development of an international control system, as well as the impact of world war.

Why change? Declining cultural acceptability; changed medical roles

Cultural positioning is an important variable underpinning the acceptability of a substance, as we can see with the changing role of cigarette smoking since the 1960s. There is some evidence that by the early years of the twentieth century, opium was less a part of everyday culture. Counter prescribing and self-medication with opium-based remedies continued, as the reminiscences of pharmacists indicate. But access to medical treatment was easier – in particular for insured workers, primarily men, after the 1911 National Health Insurance Act (NHI Act). Other drugs were favoured as more modern – aspirin and the barbiturates. In hospital practice, there was greater resistance to using opiates which were considered to be 'old fashioned', but research on medical case books has shown that their use continued to be widespread among grass-roots medical practitioners in the early decades of the century. The cultural positioning of the drug within the lay/commercial model of control was changing. We have no statistics for numbers of regular users, but the overall narcotics mortality rate was dropping. There were still regular opium-using customers in pharmacists' shops, and also a middle-class morphine-using population, generally of a higher social status. But numbers of the former were not as high as they had been.

At the same time, the role of the medical profession as a means of control was also increasingly important. Regulation by means of the prescription pad assumed enhanced importance after the 1911 NHI Act, which in general gave doctors a heightened role in terms of access to medicines. New technology also impacted on this situation. The arrival of the hypodermic syringe at mid-century was associated with the injection of morphine, the alkaloid of opium. Although hypodermic injection of the drug was by no means a medical monopoly, the profession was, via this technology, beginning to re-position its relationship to the drug. It was a significant 'gateway' for controlling medical treatment. At the same time, the emergence of theories of disease in relation to the continued use of opiates, including that of hypodermic morphine, gave the profession a dual role. Doctors were establishing control of access for the treatment of medical conditions, which needed opiates; and, at the same time, establishing the theoretical basis for seeing continued 'non-medical' use of these substances as a condition, which also required medical treatment. This medical 'British system' was emergent by the last quarter of the nineteenth century, but given heightened importance by the changed relationship between the state and the profession after the 1911 Act.

So here we have a complex of domestic issues which include both cultural positioning and the enhanced role of the medical profession, both in terms of its relationship to the state and systems of medical care, and in relation to the role of new technology and new theoretical systems and practices within the profession itself.

Opium as an international commodity: the international control system

But opium, as the discussion of trading patterns has indicated, was always more than just a national commodity. It was essential to international trading systems which were world-wide, and which could assume a political dimension, as for example during the Chinese opium wars. Recent historical work has revised earlier analyses, which stressed the 'foisting' of opium on China through the Indo-Chinese trade, and have given opium a more positive role to play in Chinese economic development. But the nineteenth-century opium wars had little impact on domestic British control systems. Of more importance was the system of Far Eastern control being discussed just before the First World War, which expanded, almost by accident, to become full-scale international control. Britain was committed before war broke out in 1914 to a system of control, which was to have a significant impact on her domestic system of regulation. A series of meetings between 1909 and 1914 laid down the bases of this system – beginning at Shanghai in 1909 and continuing at the Hague in 1911–12, 1913 and 1914. The Far Eastern opium trade was the main concern at Shanghai – moves inspired by the moral motives of American missionaries in the Philippines and by policies of extending American influence in the Pacific and extending economic influence within China. Britain had been reluctant to take part – not because of a desire to protect the Indo-Chinese trade, but through a realisation that the trade was already coming to an end and American interference was unnecessary.

But it was not America alone, but Britain and Germany who transformed a regional system into an international one. Britain and Germany, manoeuvring to protect their morphine and cocaine industries, ensured that the Hague Convention, signed in 1912, contained two crucial provisos. One was that the use of morphine and cocaine was to be confined to legitimate medical purposes; the other that no power was committed to carrying out the Convention until a world-wide list had also accepted it. These were clearly delaying tactics – which were to rebound at the end of the war. So the possibility of international control was in place by 1914, although considered unlikely at that stage. But this was to be an important and continuing issue for drug policy. Narcotics and related drugs are the only substances to be controlled at this international level. Alcohol has never been subject to international control in the same way, despite the existence of local systems of regulation in the colonies.

The impact of the First World War

The First World War was also to have a considerable impact on the way in which new systems of control were determined. The war brought about two changes important for later events – an extended system of legal regulation;

and the involvement of the Home Office, the justice ministry, as the lead government department for drug control. Two issues were involved. There was concern about the impact of lack of regulation of the supply of drugs needed for the war effort, as cocaine was smuggled to India and opium to the Far East and United States, much of it via Japan and concealed on British ships. There was anxiety also about the effects of cocaine on army efficiency, as rumours grew that the recreational use of drugs was spreading. Defence of the Realm Act regulation 40B, issued on 28 July 1916, covered cocaine, raw and powdered opium, but not morphine. Its most detailed restrictions were confined to cocaine, making it available only on prescription, to be dispensed once only. The Home Office and Sir Malcolm Delevingne, an Under Secretary who had had responsibility for drug issues there since 1913, emerged as the lead department in the negotiations round the regulation. Delevingne was a key figure in the establishment of the new 'British system', although his role there, and in the development of international control, has often been overlooked.

It was not unusual for wartime circumstances to lead to greater degrees of control than would have been feasible in times of peace. The *Lancet* recognised this in its comments at the time. The Army order which predated Regulation 40B was, it wrote, 'another instance of an innovation, long advocated in years of peace, being secured without controversy under the stimulus of a great war' (*Lancet*, 1916). War-time alcohol control provided another example. But drug control was different. Despite evidence later presented of the minute nature of the 'problem', the regulation's provisos were extended and made permanent. The 1917 report of the committee on the use of cocaine in dentistry, which investigated the extent of usage, found that 'apart from a small number of broken-down medical men' there was no evidence of much use among the general population. But these conclusions were unpopular with professional interests who wanted to extend the remit of professional control. The press, becoming at this time an independent factor in defining the issue, was more preoccupied with the image of the 'dope fiend', exemplified in its presentation of the Billie Carleton case in 1918. DORA 40B continued in operation until the Versailles peace settlement incorporated the Hague Convention of 1912. The peace settlement gave international legitimacy to the pre-war embryo system of international control.

The war established in Britain a system which was to be of great importance subsequently. It brought the Home Office into loose alliance with professional interests in medicine and pharmacy, who supported the expansion of systems of professional control. The war-time system was focused on cocaine rather than other drugs, but this was to change in the postwar period as international control was put into practice at the national level. But the penal/medical alliance which was the subsequent foundation of the British system saw its origins in events during the war.

The penal reaction to drugs in the early 1920s

This alliance had a shaky start in the early 1920s. The 1920 Dangerous Drugs Act – the British legislation which put into effect the systems of control required by the Versailles settlement – covered morphine, heroin and preparations as well as cocaine, and made provision for licensed import, manufacture, sale and distribution, provided for police inspection and laid down fines and imprisonment. But details of operation were reserved for the issue of regulations. The Act had remained a Home Office responsibility, with only a weak attempt by the newly established Ministry of Health to argue for ownership of this policy area. Soon it became obvious that Delevingne in the Home Office had an essentially short-term and penal conception of the issue. This was a question of 'stamping out addiction' through the use of police powers. Home Office regulations issued in 1921 and 1922 made it clear that professional freedoms would not stand in the way of this objective. The Home Office desire to control professionals' use of narcotic drugs raised a storm of opposition. The regulations were modified, but the following two years were marked by the intensification of a Home Office policy aimed at penalising not just addicts, but also the professionals who prescribed and dispensed to them. There were police prosecutions of pharmacists and of doctors and the Home Office was proposing that a blacklist of doctor addicts be circulated to the wholesale druggists. Another such list went to Chief Constables in 1924. Controlling maintenance prescribing by the profession was another issue; this was regarded as illegitimate by the Home Office and its chief medical adviser, Sir William Willcox. Yet many doctors were accustomed to prescribing drugs over long periods of time to users – often medical people themselves – who considered they could not function without them. The Home Office, in medical eyes, seemed to be usurping an area of the doctor–patient relationship.

The Rolleston committee and the new 'British System'

It was this situation which led to the establishment of the Rolleston committee in 1924. The nascent Home Office–medical alliance put in place during the war was under strain. The doctor–patient relationship was under threat; professional men were potential criminals; the theoretical basis of the medical role in this area – the disease view of addiction – seemed to be at risk. This was not at all what medical men had had in mind. The Home Office appeared to be attracted by penal policy initiatives in the United States, where legal moves under the 1914 Harrison Narcotics Act were criminalising doctors and pharmacists in the same way. Professor W. E. Dixon, Reader in Pharmacology at Cambridge, put the specialist view forcefully in a letter to *The Times* in 1923:

We do not seem to have learnt anything from the experience of our American brethren . . . cannot our legislators understand that our only hope of stamping out the drug addict is through the doctors, that legislation above the doctors' heads is likely to prove our undoing and that we can no more stamp out addiction by prohibition than we can stamp out insanity?

(*The Times*, 23 March 1923)

The paradox was that, although the Home Office might have wished to proceed in that way, it could not do so by itself. Doctors did have a significant role, in particular through their control of prescribing; to control them, the Home Office had to seek their support. This was what lay behind the establishment of the Rolleston committee in September 1924 as a Ministry of Health committee. The Home Office, which had initiated this move, wished to secure medical support for its position that the gradual reduction method of treating addiction was illegitimate. But there was also genuine uncertainty about which method of treating addiction was indeed proper. This move brought the Ministry of Health into an important mediating role. It might not be the lead department, but it was a major link to doctors in practice and its Regional Medical Officers had already been involved in dealing with doctor addict cases. It was a medical civil servant in the Ministry who set the revised tenor of the British system. Dr E. W. Adams, a staff medical officer, drew up in 1923 a memorandum which foreshadowed the later conclusions of the Rolleston report, of which he was the secretary. Adams combined a concern for disease views of addiction and a doctor's professional status. Thus he wrote,

if the addict is unwilling to enter into the relationship of patient to physician, but admits that he is merely coming to obtain supplies of a drug which he cannot otherwise get, then it is the clear duty of the doctor to refuse the case. But if the habitué desires treatment as a sick person for the relief of his pathological condition, the physician must be allowed to use his discretion . . .

(Ministry of Health, 1923)

Adams's view had no room at all for the old nineteenth-century lay/commercial British system.

The committee itself symbolised in its membership this medical view. All nine members and one of the two secretaries (E. W. Adams) were medical. The Chairman, Sir Humphrey Rolleston, president of the Royal College of Physicians, was an exponent of disease views of alcoholism. Professor Dixon's views have already been mentioned. His leading opponent on the committee was Willcox, the Home Office adviser, a strong supporter of institutional confinement and abrupt withdrawal for addicts, who saw addiction as in part the outcome of 'vicious causes'. The Committee was to

> consider and advise as to the circumstances, if any, in which the supply of morphine and heroin . . . to persons suffering from addiction to these drugs, may be regarded as medically advisable and as to the precautions which it is desirable that medical practitioners administering or prescribing morphine or heroin should adopt for the avoidance of excessive abuse . . .
>
> (Minute of appointment of the Committee
> (Rolleston Committee), 1926, p. 2)

In 23 meetings, with evidence from 34 witnesses, it set out a modified system of control. Most of these witnesses were also medical, like the committee itself. The Home Office attempted to structure the initial proceedings with a weighty memorandum, but the Office by no means dominated proceedings. In some ways, there was no need to, because of the enormous variation in experience and belief among the doctors called to speak to the committee. On details of policy and treatment there was variation so far as the general practitioners, consultants, Regional Medical Officers and others were concerned. Only the prison doctors formed a distinct and more homogeneous group. They always favoured harsher methods, in particular the abrupt withdrawal method of treatment; but their addict clientele was distinctly different.

The prison doctors apart, most accepted the addict's 'neurosis' and the disease view of addiction. The clientele these doctors served was middle-class, often medical itself; there was no reason therefore to jettison the disease model. This conclusion was supported in the final report which also legitimated the continuance of maintenance doses. With the exception of the prison lower-class clientele, the committee showed little interest in the consumption of other forms of opiates by other types of people. Chlorodyne, an opiate-based patent medicine, was only included in its terms of reference after a Hampstead doctor reported one of his maids found in a state of chlorodyne withdrawal. There were enough empty chlorodyne bottles in the house to fill seven pillowcases and a large wicker basket. But this type of addict was not central to the committee's interests. The committee supported the gradual withdrawal method of treatment and it opposed notification of names to the Home Office after opposition by the BMA, which regarded this as an intrusion into the doctor–patient relationship. The emphasis on those needs found significant expression in the proposal to establish a medical tribunal to police the profession. This was, as Dr Bone of the BMA put it, a means of providing 'trial by sympathetic judges'.

The final report, published in 1926, reaffirmed and developed the relationship established during the First World War. After six years of varying degrees of friction between penal and medical forms of control, both sides agreed on a system, which, although it left the Home Office in overall control, also gave professional interests considerable autonomy and power. Its publication attracted very little public attention, but its main provisos were accepted by the Home Office in amending regulations passed (after consultation with the Ministry of Health) in September 1926. Delevingne at the Home Office was thoroughly pleased with the outcome. The report was, he wrote,

> admirable and important . . . The part of the report which deals with the medical treatment of addiction and the precautions to be observed by the medical profession in connection with the administration and supply of morphine to addicts, is, I believe, the first full authoritative pronouncement on the subject, and should be a great value as a guide to the private practitioner in dealing with a very difficult class of case.
>
> (Home Office, 1926)

Impact of the report: myth and reality in the British System

The Rolleston report is widely credited with establishing something called the 'British System' of drug policy. This is generally taken to mean a system of prescribing opiates to addicts, which, in its turn, so it is argued, prevented Britain from experiencing an American-style 'war on drugs' and also the development of a drug-fuelled criminal black market. This view of Rolleston was important when reform of the American system was on the agenda in the 1960s and 1970s and when prescribing to addicts was regaining legitimacy. It has also been widely referred to in British commentary on drug policy. The real significance of the events of the 1920s was rather different. Most commentators would now agree that Rolleston was the *result* rather than the *cause* of the low numbers of addicts in Britain and their middle-class profile. Doctors who dealt with the prison population felt rather differently. If most addicts had been like the prison ones then the Rolleston report could well have taken a different stance. There was in fact no 'British system' in the way this term is often used, rather, as it has been aptly put, 'a system of masterly inactivity in the face of a non-existent problem' (Downes, 1988). Its liberalism was specific to its context not something intrinsic to British policy making. Rolleston was conceived as much in the interest of the doctor as of the addict.

But the events of the 1920s were nevertheless significant. The report was part of a more general re-ordering of relationships between professions and the developing twentieth-century state, part of Perkin's 'rise of professional society' (Perkin, 1989). It symbolised a new relationship between doctors and the state, cementing a form of regulation based on an alliance between the Home Office, the Ministry of Health and the medical profession. Doctors moved from the sidelines into a central position in policy formation. This was not, as is sometimes claimed, a medical victory but rather an accommodation of forces and realignment of the balance of power, a balance which could and would change as the profile of addiction altered. But the report cemented the fundamental alliance, which with such alteration over time, has determined and underpinned drug policy over almost 80 years. The earlier systems of regulation continued to some extent, but the primarily pharmaceutical system which had operated in the nineteenth century was no longer so central. The medico-legal alliance was henceforth dominant within policy. Although the medical input into Rolleston showed the heterogeneity of medical interest in the 1920s, the focus of the report foreshadowed subsequent psychiatric dominance of the drug addiction area. Psychiatry had an important role to play; and the conceptualisation of addiction as a middle-class neurosis underlined the speciality's move away from the asylum-based institutional options of the nineteenth century and the search for a middle-class clientele, one which 1920s addicts admirably provided. The Rolleston report has been a powerful rhetorical symbol for advocates of medical systems of drug control and for a liberalisation of prescribing. But we remember Rolleston rather than Delevingne, the Home Office civil servant, or E. W. Adams, the doctor civil servant. Arguably the relationship they symbolised was equally important. Like many such symbols, the historical reality is rather different from the myth.

References

Departmental Committee on Morphine and Heroin Addiction (1926). Report. (The Rolleston report). London, HMSO.

Downes, D. (1988). *Contrasts in Tolerance: Post-war Penal Policy in the Netherlands and in England and Wales*. Oxford, Clarendon Press.

Home Office (1926). Papers, H.O. 45/451408/27, 22 February 1926. Malcolm Delevingne's comments on the Rolleston report.

Lancet (1916). The sale of narcotic drugs to soldiers. *Lancet* 1, 475–6, 936–7, 1103–4.

Ministry of Health (1923). Papers, MH 58/275. Memorandum by Dr E. W. Adams.

Perkin, H. (1989). *The Rise of Professional Society: England since 1880*. London, Routledge.

The Times, 23 March 1923.

Chapter 3

The early years of Britain's drug situation in practice

Up to the 1960s

Bing Spear

(This chapter originally appeared in J. Strang and M. Gossop (eds) *Heroin Addiction and Drug Policy: The British System*, Oxford University Press, 1994.)

Introduction

For nearly 40 years, until the recommendations of the second Interdepartmental Committee on Drug Addiction (1965), more usually referred to as the second Brain Committee, were implemented in 1968, the British approach to the problem of opiate abuse rested on an implicit faith in the integrity of the medical profession and a wary respect for its power and influence. This was backed by a monitoring system which was at best haphazard, and at worst, non-existent.

That a loose amalgam of statutory provisions, administrative practices and professional co-operation could apparently successfully contain the level of opiate abuse in the United Kingdom, as proponents of the 'British System' claim, whilst understandable to the British, is still a topic for continuing and at times vigorous debate, analysis, misunderstanding, and deliberate distortion in those countries which traditionally have had more serious abuse problems and where rigorous regulation of professional discretion and activity is the order of the day (Spear 1975).

Whilst accepting, for the purposes of this chapter only, that there ever was, and may even still be, a special British System, it is not the intention to traverse ground which has been well traversed by others. How the 'accommodation between doctors and the Home Office in which medical involvement in strategies of control was confirmed' came into existence has been described (Bean 1974; Berridge 1984). But, as it will be some time before the official papers dealing with the changes of 1968 become available, the personal reflections of someone closely involved with events during that period may be of some interest.

The author's involvement

My involvement, as a member of the Home Office Drugs Branch Inspectorate, was during the period 1952–86, which saw two significant changes in the character and scale of the British drug abuse problem. The first of these was the emergence in the early 1950s of a small group of young heroin addicts, who differed in many respects from the heroin addicts of the pre-war period (Spear 1969); the second was the development during the 1980s of a criminal illicit traffic in heroin of a type hitherto unknown in the United Kingdom. It is with the first of these that this chapter is primarily concerned, a change which was linked to serious deficiencies in the British System. These deficiencies, were not to be rectified until 1973 and are usually ignored by those who, for various reasons, are keen to claim that the British System, or what is occasionally misrepresented as the 'British experiment with the supply of heroin to addicts', has failed. This was a fascinating, if frustrating, period made even more interesting because in 1952, when I joined the Inspectorate, its two senior members, the Chief Inspector, F. R. ('FT') Thornton, OBE, and his Deputy A. L. ('Len') Dyke, had both been involved in drug control and enforcement before the war and knew that 'scene' intimately. 'FT' had the unique distinction of having been involved since 1917 when he was transferred to the Home Office from the Board of Trade where he had been engaged in the issue of export licences for opium and cocaine under the Defence of the Realm Regulations. On the other hand Len Dyke, who held the Chief Inspector's post from 1956, when 'FT' retired, until 1965, brought a different perspective as he came to the Home Office in 1941 from the Metropolitan Police, where, as a Detective Sergeant, he had been the force's first specialist drugs officer.

The beginnings of the 'British System'

The philosophy of the British approach to the treatment of addiction can be said to have been set by the publication in 1926 of the report of the Rolleston Committee (officially the Departmental Committee on Morphine and Heroin Addiction), but the first tentative steps towards general drug control had been taken much earlier and it might be helpful to a clearer appreciation of the practical application of that philosophy if these were briefly described. In July 1916, in response to representations from the Metropolitan Police and the Service authorities about the abuse of cocaine by servicemen ('an evil, now rapidly assuming huge dimensions'), the Home Secretary was persuaded to use the special war-time powers provided by the Defence of the Realm Act to make it an offence to be in unauthorized possession of cocaine. This meant that anyone found in possession of cocaine who was not a member of the medical profession, who had not obtained the drug on a medical prescription or did not hold a permit issued by the Home Secretary, could be prosecuted for unlawful possession. Defence of the Realm Regulation 40B remained in force until replaced by the Dangerous Drugs Act 1920, and its subordinate Regulations of 1921, which extended the earlier controls to morphine and heroin. These established the broad framework of control, the basic aim of which remains today, namely the restriction of general access to 'dangerous' drugs with at the same time as little interference as possible with their legitimate use.

The 1921 Regulations authorized any medical practitioner to possess and supply drugs 'as far as may be necessary for the practice of his profession or employment in such capacity', but did not qualify that 'authority' in any way. This is important. The Regulations imposed no limitation on a doctor's choice of drug or the quantities or the circumstances under which he could prescribe; but it was assumed that he would exercise that 'authority' responsibly, in accordance with his professional judgement and the basic purpose of the legislation, which was to prevent the spread of drug addiction. This was an assumption which the Home Office soon had reason to question as evidence began to appear that doctors were supplying, or prescribing, drugs to addicts. Whether this was a proper exercise of a doctor's 'authority', and whether the supply of morphine or heroin to a person who was addicted was 'medically advisable' were questions on which the Home Office needed advice and they were accordingly referred to the Rolleston Committee with results which are well known (Bean 1974, p. 57; Judson 1974, p. 19; Trebach 1982, p. 89), if still occasionally misunderstood and misrepresented. Although the Committee's recommendations on the precautions to be observed when a patient was addicted never acquired the force of law, they were included in a revised edition of a memorandum (Home Office 1929), which was distributed to the medical and dental professions to explain the various provisions of the legislation. (Nine editions of this memorandum were prepared and distributed in the period up to 1961.)

Tribunals and scrutiny from the Home Office

Unlike Rolleston's medical recommendations, one administrative proposal, of importance in the light of the situation which was to develop 30 years later, was given legal status. This was that Tribunals should be established

> whose function it would be to consider whether or not there were sufficient medical grounds for the administration of the drugs by the doctor concerned either to a patient or to himself, and that they should advise the Home Secretary whether the doctor's right to be in possession, to administer, and to supply the drugs should be withdrawn.

The Home Secretary had had this power since 1916 under Defence of the Realm Regulation 40B in respect of authorized persons convicted of offences against the Regulations (usually of failure to maintain proper records); Rolleston proposed this should be extended to cover those medical issues which were currently causing difficulties for the Home Office.

As the argument with the recently established Ministry of Health over where responsibility for drug control should lie had been resolved in favour of the Home Office (Berridge 1984, p. 23), it fell to that Department to determine the extent to which medical practitioners were following the guidance provided by Rolleston. The primary source of information about prescribing was pharmacy records and for this the Home Office was dependent on the police. In August 1921, in a circular letter explaining the background and provisions of the recent legislation, and without apparently any prior consultation with either police, medical, or pharmaceutical interests, the Home Office requested Chief Constables to make arrangements, as part of the police's responsibility for the enforcement of the provisions relating to the supply and possession of drugs, 'for special attention to be paid to the observance of the Regulations which apply to the sales of drugs to the general public'. (The reason this responsibility was placed upon the police was quite simply that the Home Office did not itself have the resources to undertake it; in 1926, when Rolleston reported, the Home Office had only two Inspectors who were mainly preoccupied with the inspection of licensed persons and firms, the issuing of licences and the examination of statistical information about the legitimate trade.) The police were to ensure that the records and prescriptions which chemists had to keep were inspected from time to time and cases in which it was suspected that the requirements were not being observed reported to the Home Office. There was no request for regular, unusual, or large supplies to be reported, which was a serious omission not to be rectified until 1939, when a long awaited Manual of guidance included advice on the sort of information from pharmacy records which would be of interest to the Home Office.

The quiet times of the 1920s to the 1950s

The first rumblings of discontent at this new duty surfaced at the Central Conference of Chief Constables in 1925 but were firmly rejected by Sir Malcolm Delevingne of the Home Office, who made it clear that whatever the difficulties chemists should be inspected systematically. Despite this firm statement of Home Office expectations most forces took only a perfunctory interest in this duty, a level of response which was to last for some 40 years and matched an equally low level of response to the criminal aspects of drug abuse (Freemantle 1985, p. 33). Many officers regarded the inspection of pharmacy records as an extraneous duty which bore no relation to their normal police work and felt ill equipped to deal with professional men who could so easily 'blind a police officer with science'. The inadequacy of the police response was soon recognized and in 1935 Inspectors were charged with visiting all forces periodically and systematically to make certain that each had 'a staff told off for dangerous drugs work'.

For a variety of reasons, not least of which were the limited resources of the Inspectorate, the outbreak of war and the absence of any outward signs of a drug abuse problem, police interest remained at a fairly low level until the immediate postwar years when special efforts were made to revive and improve the personal liaison between the police and the Inspectorate. These efforts were gradually rewarded with an increase in the number of reports submitted to the Home Office but when I joined the Inspectorate in 1952 the overall efficiency of the inspections was still a long way short of what was desirable or acceptable and it was not until the 1980s, when specialist officers were appointed in many forces, that the standard of cover began to justify the confidence of the first Interdepartmental Committee on Drug Addiction (1961) 'that the arrangements for recording manufacture and supply, and for inspection, continue to ensure that nearly all addicts are known to the Home Office, to the Ministry of Health and to the Department of Health for Scotland' (para. 26).

The inadequate monitoring of pharmacy records probably mattered very little in the pre-war period when most of the addicts in the United Kingdom had either become addicted therapeutically and caused few problems, unlike the generation to come, or were members of the medical or associated professions, whose addiction often came to light through the Inspectorate's monitoring of wholesalers' records, as a result of their behaviour or the suspicion of a concerned pharmacist. When reports of supplies to patients were received from the police they were followed up to establish if the case was one where the drugs were required for the relief of some organic condition, in which case no further action would be taken, or if it was one of addiction, of either therapeutic or non-therapeutic origin. If the case proved to be one of addiction the rate of supply would be kept under review primarily to ensure that the prescriber was familiar with the Rolleston guidance, was not losing control of the case and was not merely pandering to the patient's addiction.

Where the supplies were ostensibly 'for practice use' it was important to confirm that they were in fact required for practice purposes and not to sustain the doctor's own addiction. Since the early days of drug control, as is shown by the unsuccessful attempt in 1922 to make it unlawful for a doctor to prescribe for himself (Berridge 1984, p. 24), the Home Office has recognized and been concerned about the special problems posed by the doctor addict. That concern was shared with the Rolleston Committee which proposed that the Home Secretary should be able to withdraw the 'authority' of such an addict on the recommendation of a medical Tribunal, which it was felt would be better able than a court of law to judge the issues involved. Although different tactics were favoured, there was clearly agreement between the Home Office and the medical profession, as represented by Rolleston, that the strategy should be to prevent doctors from using their privileged position to obtain supplies to support their own addiction and this has always been the primary objective of the Inspectorate's intervention in such cases. However, before the doctor addict could be persuaded, or in the extreme case forced by legal sanctions, to obtain their drugs from another doctor, an admission that their purchases were for their own use was desirable but, not surprisingly, was often difficult to obtain. Explanations for large or regular purchases of morphine or heroin have ranged from the unoriginal, and usually easily disproved claim that the purchaser was treating a number of terminal cases, to the much more imaginative injection of heroin into strawberry plants in the course of cancer research, and the use of heroin solutions as culture media. Although most doctor addicts could have been prosecuted for such technical offences as failing to keep, or properly maintain, a drugs register, and when convicted have had their 'authority' to possess and supply drugs withdrawn, this step was usually taken only where all other measures had failed or where the case was one in which such action was urgently necessary. For many years it was the practice to offer a doctor addict the opportunity to give a voluntary 'Undertaking', which had no legal force, that in future they would not obtain drugs for their own consumption on their own 'authority' but would obtain them from a named colleague under whose care they agreed to place themselves. This worked reasonably well, as in the case of the doctor whose longstanding Undertaking came to light only when his name was put forward in 1968 for a heroin prescribing licence, but there were also many failures although perhaps none quite as immediate as the doctor who came down from Scotland for an interview with 'FT' and on his return journey through London and Glasgow made four purchases of morphine on signed orders written on the back of his copy of the Undertaking.

New heroin addict groups begin to appear

However, in one respect the statement that nearly all addicts were known to the Home Office was correct. Since the emergence in 1951 of the new group of heroin addicts special attention had been paid by the Inspectorate to the distribution of hypodermic tablets of heroin, the form in which it was normally prescribed. This task was considerably helped by the existence in the West End of London of two pharmacies, Boots, in Piccadilly Circus, and John Bell & Croyden, in Wigmore Street, each providing a 24-hour service, and therefore very popular with addicts. Frequent inspection of the records at these two pharmacies, and the excellent co-operation of their staff, ensured that most of the addicts who were receiving heroin prescriptions quickly came to notice and the expansion of this group could be closely monitored. The arrest of 'Mark' (Judson 1974, p. 28), who had been the group's main supplier, naturally created problems. Only two of his customers had previously received prescriptions from a doctor, one used 'Mark' to supplement her prescribed supply and subsequently continued to receive prescriptions from her doctor until he decided to 'retire' in 1953. The other, a young man who had only recently come out of prison, was less fortunate as his previous prescriber, although quite willing to accept other ex-'Mark' customers, refused to take him back. However, having links with the older group of addicts he was able to persuade one of their prescribers to accept him. Only one other ex-'Mark' customer surfaced in 1951 but in 1952 eight came forward and in 1953 a further four. Given that none of these encountered any problems in finding doctors willing to prescribe for them, it is a little surprising that so many of these new addicts chose to maintain their addiction with illicit supplies, in one instance for seven years. No doubt the understandable fear, as there is today, of becoming known to authorities, a refusal to accept that they were addicted and in need of help, which receipt of a prescription would have confirmed, and the belief of many addicts that 'you don't get hooked as badly when you're buying on the black' were partly responsible for this reluctance.

If 'Mark' had introduced heroin into the West End of London where it was not currently available, the subsequent generous prescribing of a small number of doctors ensured that he would not be missed. The doctors who became involved with addicts in these early days fell into three main groups, the genuine, the gullible, and the generous, although some qualified for inclusion under more than one heading. (Ten years later gullibility and generosity were to be associated to a hitherto unrivalled extent.) Those in the first group, usually had no previous experience of addiction, tended to have only one addict patient, to maintain a firm control over a modest dosage and to do their best to persuade their patients to undergo hospital treatment. It is interesting, in view of current attitudes about the role of private prescribers, that a number of these doctors firmly believed that addicts should not be able to obtain their drugs on National Health Service (NHS) prescriptions and that a small fee was simply compensation for the trouble which addicts invariably caused. The genuinely, as distinct from the conveniently, or diplomatically gullible, formed the smallest group at this particular period and is best represented by the doctor who unhesitatingly accepted his patient's story that before taking his discharge from hospital he had been able to convince the staff he was taking only two tablets of heroin per day, whereas he actually needed a hundred each week (shortly to rise to a hundred every other day). This addict was strongly suspected of going into hospital for a partial reduction of his dosage whenever he found that his own habit was eating into his profits!

Who were the doctors?

A detailed review of the development of this new group, completed in April 1955, identified six doctors whose prescribing gave cause for concern. None of these ever had more than two or three addict patients at any one time and in 1955 only two, Dr E. A. Maguire of Linden Gardens, W2, who first came to Home Office attention in 1946 when he started to prescribe for one of the pre-war addicts, and Dr J. M. Rourke of Kensington Church Street, W8, were still actively involved. Each had only two heroin addicts and were said to have 'a working relationship', the exact nature of which was never established but which appeared to be designed to protect from prosecution those addicts who were obtaining prescriptions concurrently from each of them, sometimes on the same day. Of the others, one had decided to sever his hitherto quite extensive links with the addict world following a Court appearance in 1953, two others were successfully 'persuaded' to withdraw, whilst the oldest, who had qualified in 1903, had had no addict patients for nearly a year. This was surprising since the state of his practice suggested that any income from treating addicts was more than welcome and it was known he was not averse to telephoning a patient to enquire whether another prescription was not required.

As the following examples show, an addict accepted by any of these doctors could confidently expect his dosage of heroin to be increased virtually on request. In January 1954, Dr B who had no previous contact with addicts, began to prescribe heroin for C, a Nigerian, who claimed he had started using drugs in the USA. (Two other Nigerians who approached other doctors around the same time had been introduced to heroin by an American doctor since returned to the USA!) According to Dr B the dosage was two grains of heroin per day, yet in the first 10 days of January he gave C prescriptions for over 100 grains (6,000 mg). When asked to explain this he admitted he had merely been supplying what the addict requested and expressed his suspicion that some of the heroin was being sold. Within a short time he was prescribing cocaine in addition to heroin, again at the patient's request, C having suggested that if he were given cocaine he would be able to reduce his dosage of heroin. (Shortly afterwards the other two Nigerian addicts also asked their doctors for cocaine.) Although Dr B's practice was in North London and C had by now moved to Pimlico, he continued to treat him as a National Health Service patient, 'out of kindness' and to visit him frequently, the cost of his petrol being met by the patient. At an interview in July 1954, after which he decided to have no more dealings with addicts, Dr B again voiced his suspicions that C was selling part of his supplies in the West End at exorbitant prices. These suspicions were based on the fact that C did not work, owned two mews flats and an expensive car, and always had plenty of money. Why, if he had these suspicions, he had continued to prescribe large quantities of heroin and cocaine he could not explain, apart from saying that C had continually asked him for supplies. That Dr B was correct to regard C with some suspicion was shown by the dramatic downturn in the latter's economic situation when he came under the care of another doctor who drastically reduced, and controlled, his daily dosage.

The second example throws interesting light on the 'working arrangement' between Dr Maguire and Dr Rourke and involved another Nigerian, Broderick Walker, who in April and May 1954 endeavoured unsuccessfully to persuade six doctors that he was addicted to heroin. Nevertheless on 27 August 1954 he received his first prescription from Dr Maguire and a month later his first from Dr Rourke. Thereafter until his death in March 1955 he continued to be a patient of both doctors and in the period 27 August 1954 until 19 January 1955 received 38 NHS prescriptions from Dr Maguire for a total of 3,750 tablets of heroin and 47 NHS prescriptions for a further 3,005 tablets from Dr Rourke. On five occasions prescriptions were issued by both doctors on the same day. Although Walker claimed in an interview with police officers that he was taking six grains of heroin a day, he was in fact receiving between three and four times that amount. It is not known if at this period Dr Maguire was aware of Dr Rourke's involvement, and if so the extent of it, but there is no doubt that the latter knew Walker was a patient on Dr Maguire's NHS list as he signed some prescriptions 'pp Dr Maguire'. For a short time after Walker's death Dr Rourke continued to give prescriptions in his name to the woman with whom Walker had been living and who was also addicted. Details were submitted to the Director of Public Prosecutions and on 8 September 1955 Dr Rourke appeared at Marylebone Magistrates' Court to answer six charges of aiding and abetting the unlawful possession of drugs. Dismissing these the Magistrate, Mr Geoffrey Raphael, explained that he was 'unable to find anything (in the Regulations) which prevents a doctor exercising his own discretion and saying, "In my view this man should have this drug" and give it to him' (*Daily Telegraph*, 9 September 1955; *Criminal Law Review* 326, 1956) supporting a similar interpretation that the Regulations did not in any way limit a doctor's right to prescribe dangerous drugs, which had been given by Counsel in connection with the submission of evidence to the Rolleston Committee some 30 years earlier.

Surprisingly, Mr Raphael's decision was not interpreted by Dr Rourke as a 'green light' to expand his clientele and in the ensuing years he was content to deal with two addicts only. (Dr Maguire who had been called as a witness and had confirmed that he and Dr Rourke had a 'working arrangement' to treat each other's patients, decided that this was an opportune moment to withdraw.) Unfortunately the two addicts who remained with Dr Rourke were the two, A and D, whose names were most frequently mentioned as suppliers and the quantities of heroin they were receiving suggested the allegations were well founded. D had transferred to Dr Rourke from Dr Maguire in September 1953 and by January 1960, when he moved on to another doctor who was subsequently to prove even more generous, he was receiving around 20 grains (1,200 mg) of heroin each day. His fellow patient, A, had been accepted by Dr Rourke in January 1954 and by July was receiving a similar dosage, considerably enhanced by supplementary prescriptions which appeared to be related more to his financial circumstances than to his physical needs. (Years later A confirmed to me that he had been paying Dr Rourke between £7 and £10 per week even though he was an NHS patient.) On more than one occasion when presenting a prescription for dispensing he would have another in his hand, which he explained was 'for midnight' and by the time he transferred to another doctor in October 1958 his relationship with Dr Rourke had reached the point where he was writing his own prescriptions, merely presenting them to the doctor for signature and dating. The departure of D marked the end of Dr Rourke's involvement with addicts and he died in September 1960.

The need for a different type of response

That this was a thoroughly unsatisfactory and unacceptable state of affairs was obvious. The Inspectorate were virtually powerless, since for reasons which will shortly be explained the machinery which Rolleston had recommended to deal with such prescribing no longer existed. A very close watch was kept on what was happening and attempts were made in the course of numerous interviews with the doctors concerned to persuade them to exercise more care and control and although this was successful in two instances, Drs Maguire and Rourke proved to be totally impervious to such approaches. The police were in no better position. Although they could and from time to time did arrest addicts who were not obtaining their heroin on prescription, they were equally powerless to deal with addict-suppliers who were lawfully entitled to any heroin found in their possession. As the Head of the Metropolitan Police Drug Squad told a meeting of the Forensic Science Society in 1962, 'we have never found – or received reliable evidence – of heroin being trafficked in London in any other form than a tablet' (Cooke 1962). To prove an unlawful supply it was necessary for the police to witness the actual handover of drugs and whilst there were periods when it was possible to stand outside Boots in Piccadilly Circus and watch an addict pass on part of his recently dispensed supplies to someone else, one successful police operation there meant that future sales would be conducted under more secure conditions.

Responsibility for this situation has to rest firmly with the Home Office. As the following cases show, Drs Maguire and Rourke were not the first doctors since 1926 whose prescribing to addicts had been questionable, yet the machinery thoughtfully provided by Rolleston had never been used. Why there was such apparent reluctance to refer cases to Tribunals is not now entirely clear although there are some grounds for thinking the Home Office had quite early come to the view, later to be endorsed by the first Brain Committee, that the type of evidence likely to satisfy a Tribunal would be very difficult to obtain. (Experience gained since 1973 in using the reintroduced Tribunal machinery has shown these fears to be totally unjustified.)

In 1935 interest centred on Dr Joseph Hirshman, who in a short space of time had acquired a small group of morphine addict patients, none of whom lived in his area of London and for whom he began to prescribe. He was interviewed by Len Dyke, then still with the Metropolitan Police, who reported that in his opinion Dr Hirshman 'was one of the worst script doctors known to us' yet the relevant Home Office papers bore the cryptic comment that the Tribunal machinery, which had been introduced to deal with precisely this sort of prescribing, 'would be of little avail in the case of a man of his stamp'. Perhaps the fact that by failing to keep proper drug records Dr Hirshman had presented the Home Office with a much simpler solution had some bearing on this thinking; in February 1936 he was convicted of the technical record-keeping offence which enabled the Secretary of State to withdraw his 'authority' to possess and supply dangerous drugs. As reported in the *Morning Advertiser*,

> the importance of the prosecution was that the doctor was known to be treating a number of drug addicts and it was clear from the information in the possession of the authorities that he was not dealing with these addicts as he should. The prosecution had prescriptions to show that the doctor rather than reduce the dose of drugs, had been in a number of cases increasing the dose in a short space of a few months, one grain being increased to seven or ten grains.
>
> (*Morning Advertiser*, 26 February 1936)

Such a ready solution was not offered by Dr Gerald Quinlan who was careful not to contravene the technical requirements of the Regulations. In the immediate pre-war years Dr Quinlan collected an appreciable number of the more notorious of London's addicts and prescribed for them on a 'lavish' scale. In 1941 it was decided to approach the General Medical Council to see if they would be prepared to consider dealing with him. Again, it is not clear why the Home Office apparently did not favour reference to a Tribunal. There is little doubt the Council would have preferred to act on the basis of a conviction under the Dangerous Drugs Act but they agreed to consider the matter if the Home Office could provide evidence that Dr Quinlan had sold drugs to patients at exorbitant prices, at frequent intervals or otherwise than as medicines in the course of his treatment of them, and that, knowing they were addicted, he continued to supply them with drugs to 'their moral and physical detriment'. The facts were collected and submitted to the Council before whom Dr Quinlan was summoned to appear in June 1942. However, the hearing was repeatedly postponed and 'FT' was informed by the President of the Council that it had been intimated to him that this was a case in which the Home Office should exercise its power under the Regulations and not employ the time of a body like the General Medical Council and that he had decided to postpone the case to the November session. Not surprisingly Dr Quinlan took advantage of this breathing space and reduced both the number of his addict patients and their dosages so that when he met Len Dyke some time later he was able to claim he had 'a good defence' as he had made good progress with the addicts and had gained experience in handling them. In the circumstances the General Medical Council were informed that the Home Office would not be unduly disturbed if the case against the doctor was dropped.

Although the General Medical Council did not erase Dr Hirshman's name from the Medical Register following his conviction and were reluctant to act against Dr Quinlan, it would be wrong to give the impression that the medical authorities were entirely uninterested in the activities of such prescribers. In 1944 and in 1945 the British Medical Association and the General Medical Council enquired about the current status of the Tribunals and whether any references were likely in the near future. In reply the Home Office doubted if any useful purpose would be served by reappointing members to the Tribunal, many of whose original members had died or retired, and expressed the view that doctors who misused drugs almost invariably committed offences which could be dealt with in the Courts. This was clearly a reference to doctor addicts and was based on a review carried out in 1944 of the practice of using the Courts in such cases. (The problems posed by 'script' doctors, whose activities raised difficult questions of medical judgement, seem to have been largely ignored.) In the course of this review it was argued that the medical profession could justifiably complain that the special problems of addicted doctors were not being dealt with as Rolleston intended, but rather surprisingly the Ministry of Health took the view that doctors would prefer to be prosecuted for a technical record-keeping offence than appear before a Tribunal where the real reason for their drug purchases would be disclosed.

Within a few years the Home Office was to regret this rather negative response. The doctor concerned, Dr Marks Ripka, had first come to notice in 1935 but it was his generous prescribing in the postwar period which led to the decision in 1950 that steps had to be taken to curtail his activities. Again the preference appeared to be for proceedings in the Court, but this foundered on the same question which had caused difficulty to Sir Malcolm Delevingne in the 1920s, whether the supply of drugs to addicts could be held to be a contravention of the Regulations. It was also felt that a Court might criticize the Home Office for not referring this very difficult medical question to a Tribunal as provided for in the Regulations. As there was no reason to suppose the General Medical Council would take a different view to that taken in the case of Dr Quinlan, details of Dr Ripka's prescribing were referred to the Home Office Legal Adviser who, in February 1951, confirmed that in his view there was sufficient evidence to place before a Tribunal. The medical authorities were informed a reference was proposed and were asked to nominate members for the Tribunal. Lengthy discussions about the admissibility of evidence and a number of procedural arrangements could not be concluded until July 1952 when it was too late to include the amended provisions in the consolidated Regulations about to be introduced and it was decided these would have to be introduced separately later. However, this was not the setback it might have been because although by January 1953 Dr Ripka had accepted two of 'Mark's' former customers, his contact with this newly emerging group of addicts was about to come to an end. In February 1953 he appeared at Clerkenwell Magistrates' Court and pleaded 'guilty' to two summonses of aiding and abetting one of his patients in the unlawful possession of heroin, which she was sending to an addict then living in Malta. Dr Ripka informed the Court that he would in future accept no more addicts as patients, a welcome decision since for technical reasons the Secretary of State was unable to exercise his power to withdraw his 'authority' to possess and supply drugs (*Daily Telegraph*; *Daily Express*, 12 February 1953).

With Dr Ripka's withdrawal the re-introduction of the Tribunal provisions became less urgent but by 1955, following the review of the increasing heroin problem and the doubly unsuccessful attempt to deal with Dr Rourke, it was again clear that some control over the prescribing to addicts was necessary. (Following the dismissal of the case by Mr Raphael details of Dr Rourke's prescribing were referred to the General Medical Council who confirmed their position had not changed since 1942. In their opinion such cases should be dealt with under the appropriate provisions of the Dangerous Drugs legislation, which of course did not then exist.) Unfortunately, before the revised Regulations could be introduced the Government appointed the Committee on Administrative Tribunals and Enquiries (the Franks Committee) and it was decided the Tribunal Regulations would have to be further postponed until that enquiry had been completed. By the time the post-Franks legislation, the Tribunals and Inquiries Act 1958, was on the statute book it had been decided to review the advice given by Sir Humphrey Rolleston's Committee 30 years earlier, 'in the light of more recent developments' and the first Brain Committee was appointed in June 1958.

The first report of the Brain Committee

Their Report, published in 1961, was a classic of complacency and superficiality. The increase in the number of known addicts was simply the result of 'an intensified activity for the detection and recognition' of addiction, and there was no cause to fear that any real increase was occurring. Moreover the Committee 'were impressed' that the right of doctors in Great Britain to continue at their own professional discretion the provision of dangerous drugs to known addicts had not contributed to any increase in the total number of patients receiving regular supplies in this way. In view of this assessment of the current state of opiate abuse in the United Kingdom it is not surprising that the Committee saw no need for any significant changes in existing practices and procedures.

To criticize the Committee for their failure to recognize the change, which was then occurring, cannot just be seen as taking advantage of the power of hindsight. The threat posed by the new addicts had been accepted in 1955 by J. H. Walker, who had administrative responsibility in the Home Office for drugs policy, and would certainly have been one of the 'recent developments' placed before the Committee had he not been transferred to other work before they began their enquiry. Whilst most of the blame for the failure to bring the emergence of this new group to the attention of the Committee must rest with the Home Office, the Committee cannot entirely escape responsibility. It simply will not do to claim 'we were never told', as some members of the Committee did at the meeting of the Society for the Study of Addiction in April 1961 when 'Benny' Benjamin, the pharmacist at John Bell & Croyden, shattered the self-congratulatory atmosphere by announcing that at his pharmacy he was dispensing heroin and cocaine for more addicts than had apparently come to their notice (Judson 1974, p. 36).

The real tragedy of the first Brain Committee, however, was not the failure to recognize the new threat, serious though that was, but their naivety in believing that because they had been told (incorrectly) that there had been only two 'script' doctors in the past 20 years and their own 'widespread enquiry' had not detected the existence of Dr Rourke (who continued to prescribe for D until January 1960), there would be none in the future. Unlike their predecessors in 1926, who had had the common sense and foresight to anticipate there would probably be such cases and to suggest how they should be dealt with, all this Committee could offer was the opinion that cases of excessive prescribing were matters for the General Medical Council, an opinion which the Home Office knew, if members of the Committee did not, the Council did not share. (The reason for the Council's reluctance to get involved did not become clear until 1969 when in evidence to the Amphetamines Sub-Committee of the Advisory Committee on Drug Dependence (ACDD), the President of the Council, Lord Cohen, explained that the Council's disciplinary powers were limited to cases of 'serious professional misconduct' and that a doctor who overprescribed drugs because in good faith he regarded this as the right treatment for his patient would not be guilty of serious misconduct. It is interesting to note that the General Medical Council are now showing a far greater willingness than hitherto to test the bona fides of practitioners prescribing to addicts or drug dependents and in recent years an increasing number of doctors have been found guilty of serious professional misconduct, arising from their irresponsible or non-bona-fide prescribing.)

The second report of the Brain Committee

The cost of the first Brain Committee's failure can be seen in the dramatic rise in the number of known heroin addicts, from 62 in 1958, when the Committee was appointed, to 342 in 1964 when, as a result of two reports submitted by the Inspectorate, they were reconvened. At Lord Brain's insistence the terms of reference of this second enquiry, to review 'the advice they gave in 1961 in relation to the prescribing of addictive drugs by doctors', were deliberately narrow as the problem which the Committee was being asked to consider was clearly identified in the Inspectorate's reports. The first of these, in May 1962, was a detailed review of the prescribing of Lady I. M. Frankau, a psychiatrist of 32 Wimpole Street, in central London; the second, in November 1963, updated the special reports on the heroin problem, prepared in 1955 and 1960, and offered a number of suggestions for tackling what Judson was later to describe as prescribing of 'lunatic generosity'.

Lady Frankau

Whilst the main conclusions of this second enquiry are well known and need no further comment here, some statements in the Report have led to a serious misunderstanding of the problem the Committee faced and to the creation of a mythology which it now seems impossible to destroy or even dent. Far from being a problem of 'six' doctors, it was essentially a problem created by one, a fact readily acknowledged by Lord Brain, who after Lady Frankau had given evidence to the Committee on 4 December 1964, looked over his glasses at the civil servants at the end of the table and said, 'Well gentlemen, I think your problem can be summed up in two words, Lady Frankau.' Yet the final Report recorded that '. . . the major source of supply has been the activity of a very few doctors who have prescribed excessively for addicts' (para. 11). The reality is rather different. As Kenneth Leech, who as curate at St Anne's, Soho, was well placed to observe the developing problem, has commented,

> there never was a static group of six. At any one time between 1960 and 1968, you could identify between six and 12 doctors in the inner London area who were prescribing significant amounts of heroin for non-therapeutic purposes – that is, for addicts. The group changed from time to time, though some doctors remained constant throughout the period. In almost every case, the doctors were well-known to the Home Office drugs branch before the press discovered them.
>
> (Leech 1981)

In the original evidence to the Committee the Home Office referred anonymously to only four doctors who were prescribing, but at one of the

Committee's meetings, in reply to a member, I said I thought there were then possibly 'around six'.

This reply subsequently appeared in the Report as 'not more than six doctors have prescribed these very large amounts of dangerous drugs for individual patients . . .' (para. 12), a totally misleading statement as with one exception, all the 'very large amounts' had been prescribed by Lady Frankau. The exception, a prescription for 1,020 heroin tablets, was given to one of the veteran Canadian addicts by his NHS doctor to cover a two-week absence from London. The other 1,000-tablet prescription quoted in the Report was issued by Lady Frankau and was for 1,008 tablets of heroin and 252 grains (15,120 mg) of cocaine to cover a six-week period whilst the addict was in Wales 'withdrawing'. Instead he went immediately to Paris returning after three days to another doctor to whom he gave a different name. Lady Frankau was also the doctor responsible for the prescribing of over 600,000 heroin tablets during 1962, another of the Committee's most frequently quoted 'findings', yet the Report made no reference to the number of patients for whom this seemingly excessive quantity of drugs had been prescribed. Statistics which Lady Frankau gave to the Brain Committee showed that in the period from 1958 to 1964 she had seen just over 500 addicts which included each year about 35 who were 'not registered', undergraduates who had just started 'to play around with heroin' and about 30 old cases. On a list which she gave me in 1966, for the purpose of a follow-up study which because of her subsequent illness was never completed, there were 374 names, the vast majority of whom were heroin addicts for whom she had prescribed and whose prescriptions had been traced. (This list showed that in 1962 she had accepted, and prescribed for, 74 new addict patients compared with 125 in the statistics given to the Brain Committee.)

As Lady Frankau's prescribing was undoubtedly the mainstay of the flourishing illicit market in heroin and cocaine in London until 1966, some comment on her treatment philosophy and methods is necessary. Her interest in the treatment of drug addiction appears to have been first aroused towards the end of 1957 when Dr P. M. Stanwell, a general practitioner who already had one or two addict patients, suggested to her in the course of a consultation about an alcoholic that she might like to try her hand with an addict, but it was not until the following summer that the extent of this interest became apparent. This was because all the prescriptions were written by Dr Stanwell with Lady Frankau providing supportive psychotherapy as a preliminary to the addicts undergoing withdrawal treatment in a nursing home under her supervision. Gradually the number of patients being accepted for treatment increased, with Lady Frankau more directly involved in the issue of prescriptions, a development which eventually led to a break with Dr Stanwell who had become very concerned at Lady Frankau's readiness to increase an addict's dosage on the flimsiest of pretexts, whilst Lady Frankau, for her part, believed that Dr Stanwell was far too firm.

The effect of the removal of such restraining influence as Dr Stanwell had been able to exercise was soon apparent as Lady Frankau's prescribing became increasingly bizarre and irresponsible. The more startling examples of her prescribing have been quoted in the second Brain report and while there are many more which could be given, it is the rationale behind this prescribing (Frankau and Stanwell 1960) which is of interest. Put simply, the essential element of Lady Frankau's treatment philosophy was that the patient had to be made independent of the illicit market, although in many instances the practical effect was merely to change the addict's role in relation to the market, from customer to supplier. One of the difficulties in achieving this independence was the addicts' inability

> to say simply that they had overstepped the usual amount, instead they either augmented their supplies from the black market, or produced plausible stories of accidents or losses. Eventually they realised that it was better to state bluntly that too much had been used. Extra supplies were prescribed to prevent them returning to the black market, which would involve them in financial difficulties, and (which is even more important) would mean a return to the degradation and humiliation of contacting the pedlars . . . During this phase of treatment the addicts acquired enough insight into their condition to be able to cooperate.
>
> (Frankau and Stanwell 1960)

This was amplified in her Niagara Falls address in February 1963 when she explained that each patient

> was assured that prescriptions would always be available and, that if he could genuinely claim to have spilled or lost part of his supply, the lost drug would be replaced. If he had used too much and came and reported this, he would be given a prescription and the reasons for his lapse be discussed.
>
> (Frankau 1964)

Clearly the success of such a policy rested upon the ability to determine whether claims for additional or replacement supplies were genuine and it was in this respect that Lady Frankau clearly had a distinct advantage over other doctors since, as she frequently asserted, she could always tell if one of her patients was lying. Her willingness to entertain such claims confirmed the ingenuousness first hinted at in the 1960 paper and which no doubt partly accounted for the irregularity of her prescribing, where not only the interval between prescriptions varied widely but so also did the quantities prescribed and it was not uncommon to find two, or even three, prescriptions to the same addict dispensed on the same day. To this ingenuousness has to be added an unrivalled capacity for self-deception (typified by her statement to the Brain Committee that 'all my patients are too tightly controlled to sell drugs on the black market'), which in its turn led to an unshakeable confidence in the correctness of her methods and a haughty intolerance of other approaches and disregard for many of the normal courtesies of medical practice. These attributes are well illustrated by a case involving a patient who was convicted of obtaining 'dual supplies' of heroin concurrently from Lady Frankau and his NHS general practitioner, who had written to her for a report but had had no reply. When first told she would be required to attend Court Lady Frankau complained to the Home Office that she did not have the time as 21 patients were scheduled to come for their prescriptions between 10 a.m. and 11 a.m. on the morning of the hearing (an average of three minutes per consultation). In Court she said she had a large number of addicts as patients and had no time to write or talk to any doctor; she had asked the addict if he was still going to his general practitioner and accepted his reply that he was not. The addict's version was that when his NHS doctor went on holiday he simply went to Lady Frankau who gave him 'large supplies': 'I just asked for what I wanted and she took my word. If you spun her enough story she would believe you.'

Of the many myths to which this period has given birth three of the most persistent are that the 'six' were all in private practice, that the influx of Canadian, and to a lesser extent US, heroin addicts in the early 1960s was the direct result of a lecture tour which Lady Frankau made to Canada and that her involvement with addicts was motivated entirely by financial considerations. All are wrong. Although the second Brain Report offered no information on the point, Lady Frankau was the only private prescriber at that time and the concern expressed in para. 7.13 of the 'Treatment and Rehabilitation' Report of the Advisory Council on the Misuse of Drugs (1982) was shared by the 1960s prescribers. Their attitude to this delicate question was fairly reflected in Dr Hawes' comment that 'to have accepted any as private patients would have laid one open to the charge of having a vested interest in addiction' (Hawes 1970).

The Canadians

As has been shown (Spear and Glatt 1971; Zacune 1971), the peak of the Canadian influx was in 1962, a year before Lady Frankau gave her paper at Niagara Falls and her own records show that in 1962 she accepted 26 new addicts from Canada but only six in the following year and 13 in 1964. Whilst her visit to Canada inevitably attracted considerable press attention, what those who have chosen to represent it as a recruiting drive have failed to appreciate is the effectiveness of the addicts' grape-vine, which had already relayed back to Canada the experiences of the first arrivals, who had found the United Kingdom, with its readily available supplies of legitimate heroin, to be the 'seventh heaven' they had been led to believe. This invasion had little effect on an indigenous situation which had been developing steadily since 1951, without trans-Atlantic help and its limited extent was predicted with remarkable accuracy by the then RCMP Liaison Officer in London.

Just as the influence of Canadian addicts on the domestic heroin scene has been exaggerated, so too has been the influence of US addicts and again it is Lady Frankau's involvement with this group which has received most attention. The number of US addicts for whom she prescribed during the period 1958 to 1966 was about 60, few of whom were long-term residents. The largest number of new cases (20) occurred in 1965 by which time, as word passed along the addicts' grape-vine, she had acquired a considerable international reputation as an unquestioning supplier of drugs. It was well known in addict circles in Paris that in times of need supplies of heroin could always be obtained by the simple expedient of visiting Lady Frankau, and admirably demonstrated by one internationally famous jazz musician who arrived at London Airport from Paris one morning in March 1962 and departed the same afternoon after receiving from Lady Frankau a prescription for heroin, cocaine, and methadone.

Of the many reasons which have been advanced to explain Lady Frankau's involvement the one for which there is no evidence is that she was financially motivated and allegations that she was can usually be traced to disgruntled addicts or to doctors unable to accept that anyone would willingly devote so much time trying to help such undeserving cases without adequate financial reward. In fact from the outset, her work with addicts was subsidized by her private psychiatric practice and it was by no means uncommon at West End pharmacies to find prescriptions endorsed 'charge to my account'. Whilst many of her critics preferred to keep their distance, those, including some of her severest, who did meet her to discuss her treatment philosophy and methods, invariably admitted afterwards that although she might be misguided, or in the words of one, be 'a well meaning fool', her sincerity and integrity could not be doubted.

That these and other myths should still exist after so many years is regrettable as they give a misleading picture of a critical period in the development of the British drug problem, a period which saw fundamental changes in both the character and extent of that problem. Yet these changes continue to be represented as the result of the activities of a few rogue or misguided doctors, an analysis which if understandable in the 1960s, is not today. We had moved from a reasonably comfortable situation in which the typical addict was 'a middle aged housewife whose illness was treated if not understood, with some measure of success by the family doctor', to one in which 'the known mores of pre-war surburbia were exchanged for those of a youthful minority subculture of the Western World' and in which 'the comforting solidity of expert ignorance was exchanged for the frightening limbo of a world where each expert's word contradicted that of the next' (Home Office Drugs Branch 1968). It was a situation for which we were not prepared.

It is therefore not surprising that the temptation to ignore the significance of what was really happening, and to place responsibility for these changes on a few readily identifiable scapegoats, could not be resisted. The blanket criticism of all the 1960s prescribers, apart from being grossly unfair, diverts attention from the real tragedy of the period, the unwillingness of the vast majority of the medical profession to take up the challenge which these new young addicts presented. Any doctor who ventured into this area, and most chose not to, had to be 'unusually brave, compassionate, skilful and lucky if he were to achieve success' and there is no doubt that most of those who did become involved were dedicated practitioners who were prepared to put themselves to endless trouble on behalf of the addicts (Jeffery 1970). The *Sunday Times*, following an investigation in which the main prescribers were interviewed 'at length', concluded that

> all of these doctors have some unusual quality about them – some direct element of the 'outsider' in their make-up; strong political opinions; the status of exile; or perhaps an unusual degree of professional compassion. And it is possible as a result of this that they succeed in acting as a link between the outcast addicts and normal society.
>
> (*Sunday Times*, 20 February 1966)

Unfortunately, the fact that only a handful were prepared to respond to the new challenge meant that they did not have the necessary time to decide which were reasonable demands and which were not. In the words of Dr Hawes:

> you became a junkie doctor with one patient; if you responded to his plea you had started your career in that line, because he sent his friends and they sent their friends. Soon you would be (as I was) overwhelmed by the sheer numbers. In the past ten years I had through my hands (not treated) somewhere about a thousand addicts. I kept fairly full notes about the first three hundred, but after that time allowed no more than the bare details.
>
> (Hawes 1970, pp. 258–60)

Moreover, those who were prepared to help quickly found that the kind of assistance from hospital out-patient and in-patient services, upon which general practitioners could ordinarily rely, was 'almost totally lacking' when the patients were addicts (Hewetson and Ollendorff 1964).

Non-participation from the majority of doctors

If further confirmation was needed that the vast majority of United Kingdom doctors wanted as little contact as possible with addicts, a situation which

has changed little over the past 35 years, it is provided by their response to
the Brain II proposals. Ten years earlier the profession had rightly, vigor-
ously and successfully, resisted the Government's plan to ban the future
production and use of heroin (Bean 1974, p. 133; Judson 1974, p. 29), yet
the imminent limitation on the hitherto unfettered, and jealously guarded,
right of a doctor to prescribe whatever drug he considered to be in his
patient's best interest, attracted very little discussion or opposition. Reasons
for this uncharacteristic response are not hard to find. First, as Glatt *et al.*
have suggested, there was an ideological objection because

> addicts have a very poor prognosis, and basic to the ideology of most
> doctors is that they should attempt to cure their patients. This of course
> means that the doctor must first accept the idea that drug addiction is
> a disease and treatable in general practice. It would seem that this idea
> is not yet accepted by many British doctors . . .
>
> (Glatt *et al.* 1967)

Second, the new arrangements would give general practitioners in particular,
protection from the kind of pressures described by Dr Hawes; a doctor
who did not have the legal right to prescribe heroin was far less likely to be
approached for 'treatment'. The removal of a power which had never been
used was likely to excite only those doctors who saw the matter as an issue
of principle and a campaign to preserve an unfettered freedom to prescribe
heroin to addicts was unlikely to attract much support from a public which
had been left in little doubt by the publicity given to the 'six', and to the
later activities of Dr John Petro and Dr Christopher Swan (Judson 1974,
p. 58; Leech 1981; Trebach 1982, p. 178; Freemantle 1985, p. 23), that the
current heroin problem was largely the result of that unfettered freedom.

Whilst the negative response of the medical profession is perhaps understandable, the Brain II proposals, and their implementation, have not escaped
criticism entirely. If Brain II had 'narrowed the problem down to only a
few doctors, why did the medical profession and the government not proceed to deal with those few?' (Trebach 1982, p. 117) and what were 'the
serious matters involving extensive consultation "as professional interests"
were involved' which meant that it took over two-and-a-half years to implement the Committee's findings? (Bean 1974, p. 83). These questions will
not be satisfactorily answered until the relevant Ministry of Health papers
are released but it was apparent at a very early stage in the Committee's
deliberations that not only did they still hold the view, expressed in their
first Report (para. 44) that special Tribunals would be difficult to establish,
but they were very much attracted to the concept of special centres at which
addicts could be treated. (The suggestion that a speedy reintroduction of
updated Tribunal machinery, possibly linked to some statutory limitation
on the number of addicts an individual doctor could treat, and the maximum

dosage which could be prescribed without a second opinion, did not find much support.) As the idea of special treatment centres had been put forward by one of the psychiatrist witnesses (Bewley 1965) and the Report suggested that such centres 'might form part of a psychiatric hospital or of the psychiatric wing of a general hospital' (para. 22), the 'psychiatrizing' of addiction treatment policy in the United Kingdom was assured.

Given that this was the chosen, and accepted, solution to the problem of the over-prescriber, the delay in the implementation of the proposals was inevitable. Existing facilities were clearly inadequate and would be unable to cope with the numbers of addicts who would have to be transferred from the general practitioners currently looking after them, let alone those who, it was hoped, would be encouraged to quit the illicit market. With few exceptions most psychiatrists had successfully avoided, or had had little opportunity for contact with these young addicts and consequently had very little practical experience upon which to draw, whilst those doctors with such experience, the heavily criticized general practitioners, were to be denied further involvement. It was not surprising therefore that the influence of US thinking did not take long to surface. An early proposal, unveiled at a meeting at the Home Office, was that the prescribing of heroin would be discontinued despite the very clearly expressed view of Brain II (para. 15) that addicts should be able to obtain supplies of this drug 'from legitimate sources'. Although this proposal was dropped in the face of strong Inspectorate objections, the advocates of a methadone-only, and an eventual non-prescribing policy, were to obtain their objective, by other means.

Those responsible for planning the new centres had been given no detailed blueprint by Brain II but they were fortunate to be able to draw on the experience of Dr John Owens at All Saints Hospital, Birmingham, who in 1964 had established an addiction unit, which over the next two years attracted increasing numbers of young heroin addicts. Some of these were self-, some medical, referrals, but significant numbers were referred by the police and probation services. The All Saints approach, embodying those same principles, controls on prescribing, responsible behaviour by the addicts and good relations with the community, which led Connell to exempt the Shreveport clinic of Dr Butler from his general criticism of the failed American clinics of the 1920s (Trebach 1982, p. 187), successfully contained the problem in the Birmingham area and has not received the recognition it deserves (Nyman 1969; Judson 1974, p. 88).

Whether, as is sometimes suggested, the delay in phasing out the prescribing general practitioners, and the uncertainty 'on the street' about what was going to happen contributed significantly to the way in which the United Kingdom heroin problem was to develop, is for social historians of the future to determine. What is certain is that during this period two important barriers came down. First, the reluctance of an addict population, which up until then had been almost entirely dependent on pharmaceutical heroin, to use illicitly manufactured heroin of unknown purity and strength, gradually disappeared and 'Chinese' heroin became a regular feature of the London black market. Second, early in 1968, largely through the efforts of Dr Petro, the amount of injectable methyl-amphetamine in the West End of London increased dramatically and, as Leech (1973) has described, 'provided the bridge between the needle culture and the kids in the clubs' making 'the process of "fixing" an integral part of the West End drug culture', and to transform it over the next few years into a multi-drug injecting 'scene'. The inadequacies of the existing legislation, and the continuing absence of effective machinery to deal with dubious prescribing, which were not to be rectified until 1973, ensured there were sufficient supplies of methadone, amphetamines, methylphenidate ('Ritalin'), barbiturates, and dipipanone ('Diconal'; later to become a sufficiently serious problem to justify it being placed under the same prescribing restrictions as heroin and cocaine), to supplement the dwindling supplies of heroin from the treatment centres (Spear 1982).

Conclusion

It could be said that the 'British System', as it evolved following Rolleston, ceased to exist in 1953, when the Tribunal provisions were dropped, but it is the restrictions on prescribing which came into effect on 16 April 1968 which have been interpreted as heralding the end of the Rolleston era and the formal abandonment of the British System. This is a total misreading of the situation, which first overlooks the fact that the 1968 changes were a response to a specific problem, the prescribing of heroin and cocaine by one doctor. They were not intended to replace the advice given by the first Brain Committee which had reviewed the general addiction problem a few years earlier and endorsed the Rolleston concept of 'the stabilised addict' (para. 36). The basic philosophy of the British approach was unaffected by the 1968 changes and currently, an addict to heroin, or any other drug, is as free to consult any doctor of his choice, and for that doctor to accept or reject him, as would have been the case in 1926. The only difference is that the doctor would now be unable to prescribe heroin, cocaine, or dipipanone unless specially licensed but would be perfectly entitled to give his patient any other drug for the purpose of 'maintenance', 'stabilization' or in the course of a detoxification regimen. The decision whether or not to issue a licence rests with the Home Secretary, after consultation with the Department of Health, and whilst it is current policy not to license general practitioners to prescribe heroin, there is nothing in the Regulations to prevent a general practitioner from applying for a licence, and if refused, from challenging that decision in the Courts. (A few licences to prescribe dipipanone have in fact been issued to general practitioners.)

The belief that the British System has now been abandoned arises from a misunderstanding of the relationship between the law and the conduct of medical practice. As mentioned above, United Kingdom drug laws aim to provide a framework within which doctors are free to use drugs in accordance with their clinical judgement, which may or may not accord with the consensus of medical opinion at that time. Whether a particular drug is used in the treatment of a specific disease is not a matter to be dictated by the Department of Health, the Home Office, or any other government agency, a fact still not fully appreciated even in this country. What is now being interpreted as the formal abandonment of the British System is merely a change in medical attitudes which Fazey has ascribed to the seizure of the moral high ground by a group within the medical establishment and psychiatry in particular,

> who declared unilaterally that drug addicts should not be given drugs . . . Psychiatrists who took over treatment decided that the U.S.A. knew best, and addicts could be cured of their addiction. Abstinence became the universal goal to be enforced by only offering detoxification regimes, as in-patients or out-patients and oral methadone in a few cases.
>
> (Fazey 1989)

This shifting of the goalposts away from the clearly expressed intention in 1968 that heroin should still be supplied in minimum quantities 'to avoid the development of an organized illicit traffic on a scale hitherto unknown in this country', and that the out-patient clinics would make 'drugs available to those addicts who could not be persuaded to do without them' (Ministry of Health 1967; Glancy 1972) was not based on a proper evaluation of previous policies. Moreover, this change was accompanied by pressure to conform to the new orthodoxy, which in 1984 was enshrined in 'Guidelines of good clinical practice in the treatment of drug misuse' (Department of Health 1984), drawn up by a working group of doctors with expertise in the field, mainly psychiatrists, and representatives of various medical bodies. As these guidelines were distributed by the Department of Health to all doctors, it is understandable that they should be seen as 'official' discouragement to any doctor still favouring the Rolleston approach, and effectively ensure the virtual, universal acceptance of the new orthodoxy.

However, the advent of AIDS has introduced a new element into the equation and the validity of such an inflexible non-prescribing approach, in the face of a threat which has been officially recognized as posing a greater danger to public health than drug misuse (Advisory Council on the Misuse of Drugs 1988) is now being seriously questioned. The next few years may therefore see at least a partial return to principles and practices which were jettisoned for medico-political reasons before they had been properly tested or evaluated and not because they had failed. It would therefore be premature to write the obituary of the British System; it has merely been under psychiatric care for the past 35 years.

References

Advisory Committee on Drug Dependence (1970). The amphetamines and lysergic acid diethylamide. HMSO, London.

Advisory Council on the Misuse of Drugs (1982). Treatment and rehabilitation. HMSO, London.

Advisory Council on the Misuse of Drugs (1988). AIDS and drug misuse. HMSO, London.

Bean, P. (1974). *The social control of drugs*. Martin Robertson, London.

Berridge, V. (1984). Drugs and social policy: the establishment of drug control in Britain 1900–1930. *British Journal of Addiction*, 79, 18–29.

Bewley, T. H. (1965). Heroin and cocaine addiction. *Lancet*, 1, 808–10.

Cooke, E. (1962). The drug squad. *Journal of the Forensic Science Society*, 3, 43–8.

Departmental Committee on Morphine and Heroin Addiction (1926). Report. (The Rolleston Report.) HMSO, London.

Department of Health (1984). Guidelines on good clinical practice in the treatment of drug misuse. HMSO, London.

Fazey, C. S. J. (1989). What works: an evaluation of drug treatments for illicit drug users in the United Kingdom and Europe. Studies of Drug Issues: Report No. 3. Centre for Urban Studies, University of Liverpool.

Frankau, I. M. (1964). Treatment in England of Canadian patients addicted to narcotic drugs. *Canadian Medical Association Journal*, 90, 421–4.

Frankau, I. M. and Stanwell, P. M. (1960). The treatment of drug addiction. *Lancet*, December, 1377–9.

Freemantle, B. (1985). *The fix*. Michael Joseph, London.

Glancy, J. E. McA. (1972). The treatment of narcotic dependence in the United Kingdom. *Bulletin on Narcotics*, XXIV, 4, 1–9.

Glatt, M. M., Pittman, D. J., Gillespie, D. G. and Hills, D. R. (1967). *The drug scene in Great Britain*. Edward Arnold, London.

Hawes, A. J. (1970). Goodbye junkies – A general practitioner takes leave of his addicts. *Lancet*, 2, 258–60.

Hewetson, J. and Ollendorff, R. H. V. (1964). Preliminary survey of one hundred London heroin and cocaine addicts. *British Journal of Addiction*, 60, 109–14.

Home Office (1929). Memorandum as to duties of doctors and dentists. HMSO, London.

Home Office Drugs Branch (1968). The dangerous drugs legislation, 1967. *The Police Journal*, LXI, 249–54.

Interdepartmental Committee on Drug Addiction (1965). Second Report. (Second Brain Report.) HMSO, London.

Jeffery, C. G. (1970). *In: Modern trends in drug dependence and alcoholism*. Butterworths, London.

Judson, H. F. (1974). *Heroin addiction in Britain*. Harcourt Brace Jovanovich, New York and London.

Leech, K. (1973). *Keep the faith baby*. SPCK, London.

Leech, K. (1981). John Petro, the junkies' doctor. *New Society*, 56(969), 430–2.

Ministry of Health (1967). The treatment and supervision of heroin addiction. Hospital Memorandum [67], 16.

Nyman, M. (1969). Addiction unit, All Saints' Hospital. *British Journal and Social Service Review*, August, 1451–2.

Spear, H. B. (1969). The growth of heroin addiction in the United Kingdom. *British Journal of Addiction*, 64, 245–56.

Spear, H. B. (1975). The British experience. *The John Marshall Journal of Practice and Procedure*, 9, 67–98.

Spear, H. B. (1982). *In: The dependence phenomenon*. MTP Press, Lancaster.

Spear, H. B. and Glatt, M. M. (1971). The influence of Canadian addicts on heroin addiction in the United Kingdom. *British Journal of Addiction*, 66, 141–9.

Trebach, A. S. (1982). *The heroin solution*. Yale University Press, New Haven.

Waller, T. (1990). Ways to open the surgery door. *Druglink*, 5(3), 10–11.

Zacune, J. (1971). A comparison of Canadian narcotic addicts in Great Britain and in Canada. *Bulletin on Narcotics*, XXIII, 4, 41–9.

Chapter 4

The drugs problem of the 1960s

A new type of problem

Thomas Bewley

Introduction

Before the 1960s there were only two known types of drug dependence in Britain. Dependence on Alcohol and Dependence on Tobacco. There was little interest in dependence on alcohol, though there was an awareness that some people drank excessively and that this could be damaging. There was no real public awareness that tobacco (nicotine) caused dependence or addiction. Nor was there much accurate knowledge of the many harms to health caused by its consumption. At this time there was virtually no 'non-therapeutic' use of drugs of any sort, whether drugs had been obtained illicitly, or by diversion of some medications obtained on prescription. There was also very little awareness either by the public, or by the medical profession, that many drugs, both sedatives and stimulants, could lead to dependent use. The commonsense view at that time was that there were only a handful of patients dependent on drugs, being those addicted to opiates initially prescribed for medical treatment.

All this changed markedly in the 1960s. Public concerns were raised by the knowledge that many young people had begun to experiment with drugs of different types such as cannabis, opiates, amphetamines and other stimulants as well as hallucinogens such as LSD. This led to the setting up of various committees which reported and made recommendations. The Brain committee reported on opiates (and cocaine) twice and the Wootton Committee reported on cannabis. These reports suggested guidelines to deal with what was perceived to be a new problem. They have been the basis for dealing with all such problems up to the present day (Ministry of Health 1961, 1965; Home Office 1968). This was also the decade when patterns of smoking began to change (Doll and Hill 1964) and over which consumption of alcohol continued to rise (Brewers and Licensed Retailers 1980).

Following the end of the Second World War in 1945 there were changes in many countries with the start of increased affluence and increased travel between them. There was also much greater knowledge of what happened in other parts of the world. All of this made an increase in the use of psychoactive substances for recreational purposes inevitable. The speed of change varied from country to country and was clearly seen in the 1960s in England. Because there had been virtually no problems with drugs of any sort earlier there was no guidance on the best methods of dealing with the problems. In the early 1960s there had been little evidence of smuggling of opiates and it would appear that most of the newly notified addicts had obtained their drugs initially from others, who had themselves had had drugs prescribed for them. With the benefit of hindsight it would appear that the level of prescribing made it possible for addicts to use only some of the drugs prescribed for them for themselves. As well as this, they were able to give, lend, share or sell the remainder of the drugs prescribed for themselves to others.

Opiates

In the 1960s it became clear that there had been a change in the type of opiate addict notified to the Home Office. A small number of addicts who had become dependent on heroin obtained illicitly were reported to the Home Office for the first time. The number of these non-therapeutic addicts rapidly increased. The numbers of therapeutic addicts hardly changed at all (Bewley 1965a, b). At this time also a small number of slightly older non-therapeutic heroin addicts arrived from Canada for private treatment by Dr I. M. Frankau (Lady Frankau, the wife of Sir Claud Frankau, Consultant Surgeon, St George's Hospital). Twenty-six such addicts arrived in 1962 but the numbers each year diminished rapidly in the next five years (Frankau 1961, 1964).

There were two reports from an Interdepartmental Committee which was chaired by Sir Russell (later Lord) Brain, the President of the Royal College of Physicians of London (Ministry of Health 1961, 1965). The first report in effect decided that the guidelines laid down in the Rolleston Commission of 1926 were satisfactory and that there was no need to make any changes. Unfortunately the Committee had merely looked at the total numbers of opiate addicts known to the Home Office each year which had changed little. A closer look would have shown that while the number of therapeutic addicts was decreasing the number of non-therapeutic addicts was doubling every 18 months. This became very clear in the 1960s (see Table 4.1). Shortly before the publication of the first report, Sir Russell Brain spoke to the Society for the Study of Addiction in an anodyne way, but was embarrassed when Mr Benjamin, a pharmacist, said that he saw in John Bell & Croyden's chemist shop each week considerably more addicts than the Committee were apparently aware of. As well as this he had seen a new addict with an enormous prescription for heroin and cocaine and could only assume he must have become addicted by getting drugs from other addicts in large amounts as there were no other sources of supply. Sir Russell could only reply that if

Table 4.1 The increase of non-therapeutic heroin addicts in the 1960s

Year	No. of new non-therapeutic heroin addicts
1960	23
1961	54
1962	72
1963	90
1964	160
1965	258
1966	518
1967	745
1968	1304

Source: Home Office: Annual Reports, 1960–1968.

that was the case nobody had told them (Brain 1961). It soon became obvious that the first committee report had been wrong and that the committee would have to be recalled (Bewley 1964). Sir Russell however ensured that the remit for the recalled committee would solely cover doctors' prescribing. (The committee had also produced an interim report dealing with the problems of anaesthetists who sniffed anaesthetic gases (Ministry of Health 1959).) The second report appeared in 1965 and made a set of recommendations closely following those in an article in the *Lancet* (Bewley 1965a, b, 1968b). This article was a shortened version of a memorandum written for the Committee. The recommendations were that there should be controls over the prescribing of opiates to addicts. There should be special centres to deal with the problem. There should be a standing advisory committee to review progress. There should be a formal notification system.

In the 1960s drug dependence was a new phenomenon. The majority of addicts were young and had relatively short histories of dependence. Unlike the United States there were very few elderly addicts who had had problems for many years. This led to a vague hope that somehow with vigorous action 'drugs' would go away and we all would be back in the halcyon previous days when addiction hardly existed at all. A comparison of the United States scene with that of Britain drew attention to the problems of chronicity and the need to care for those with problems who did not recover (Bewley 1969a). It was at this time that it was necessary to consider other aspects of the problem such as harm reduction. A study of the self-injecting techniques of addicts showed that much that was happening was filthy, unsanitary and unsafe (Bewley 1968a, b, c). Those treating addicts in the mid-1960s began to counsel addicts on safe injection techniques and started in a small way supplying sterile syringes which later became formally institutionised in needle exchange schemes (Bewley 1975).

Another curious artefact during this decade was an enormous interest in what became widely known, particularly in the USA, as the 'British System'. This was a curious idea that somehow in England, because opiates could be freely prescribed for addicts, the whole problem of addiction had been solved and would rapidly go away (Bewley *et al.* 1972; Brown 1915). Many comparisons were made with the situation in the United States where prescribing opiates was not possible till Vincent Dole introduced the prescribing of methadone (Dole *et al.* 1967).

Cocaine

In the 1960s there was very little use of cocaine except by a single group – opiate addicts who had cocaine prescribed for them by the doctors who prescribed heroin for them. There was no scientific reason for this but the practice was to prescribe about two-thirds of the dose of heroin as the dose of cocaine. New addicts would arrive at a doctor announcing 'I am a 6 and 4' or 'I am a 10 and 7' referring to a number of grains of heroin and cocaine they expected to be prescribed for them. There was virtually no cocaine smuggled into the country and then sold for recreational purposes. No one had heard of Colombian cocaine cartels, and 'crack' was a future that no one thought about at that time.

Cannabis

Because of concern about the increase in the use of cannabis the Government's Standing (Interdepartmental) Advisory Committee on Drug Dependence set up a subcommittee chaired by Baroness Wootton to prepare a report (Home Office 1968). This was generally referred to as 'the Wootton report' after its chairman. The Committee reviewed the international background with an appendix explaining how cannabis had been included with opiates in the treaties that preceded the International Opium Convention. The committee reviewed the effects of cannabis in different countries including its possible therapeutic uses, the place of cannabis in the United Kingdom drug scene and the existing provisions for controlling the drug under the dangerous drugs Acts. One section of the report considered the social aspects of cannabis use and the controversy about its dangers, particularly the claims that its use led to either opiate addiction or to violent crime. Attention was paid to a review of the salient literature on these topics and this was presented fully in an appendix. As far as progression to heroin use was concerned the subcommittee concluded that the risk of progression to heroin from cannabis was not a reason for retaining control over the drug. As far as progression to crime was concerned they thought that excessive use of cannabis might lead to an attack of disturbed consciousness, excitement, agitation or panic and reduced self-control. The extent to which the affected person might commit a violent crime would depend more on his personality than on the amount of cannabis he had taken. The link with violent crime was obviously greater with alcohol, and in the United Kingdom the taking of cannabis 'had not, so far, been regarded even by its severest critics as a direct cause of serious crime'. Another section was a comparison of cannabis and other drugs consisting of a comparison between the effects of cannabis and the effects of barbiturates, minor tranquillisers, alcohol and tobacco. In this section the committee pointed out that to make comparative evaluation between cannabis and other drugs was to venture into highly subjective territory.

The committee stated that the evidence before them showed: An increasing number of mainly young people, in all classes of society, were experimenting with the drug and substantial numbers used it regularly for social pleasure. There was no evidence that this activity was causing violent crime or aggressive antisocial behaviour or was producing in otherwise normal people conditions of dependence or psychosis requiring medical treatment. The experience of other countries was that once it was established, cannabis smoking tended to spread. In some parts of Western society where interest in mood-altering drugs was growing there were indications that it might become a functional equivalent of alcohol. In spite of the threat of severe penalties and considerable effort at enforcement the use of cannabis in the United Kingdom did not appear to be diminishing. There was a body of opinion that criticised the legislative treatment of cannabis on the grounds that it exaggerated the dangers of the drug and needlessly interfered with civil liberty. A full-page advertisement in *The Times* newspaper on Monday 24 July 1967 drew attention to the problems of cannabis use with a statement, 'The law against marijuana is immoral in principle and unworkable in practice.' This was signed by 64 members of the great and good. The Wootton committee however concluded that in the interests of public health it was necessary to maintain restrictions on the availability and use of the drug. For the purpose of enforcing restrictions, the committee saw no alternative to the criminal law and its penalties. They discussed the arguments in favour of legalisation of cannabis but ruled them out for the near future. When the report was published it was generally attacked as being 'soft on drugs' but over time it came to be seen as a sensible report and its recommendations have been accepted and there followed a progressive lowering of penalties in practice over the following 30 years (Bewley 1969b).

Amphetamines

In the 1960s another change to occur was the realisation that amphetamines could be addictive. Amphetamines had been widely used during the Second World War to help pilots to remain alert and awake. Following the war these were much used in medicine to treat depression. They were believed to be a safe non-addictive drug. In 1954 (Ministry of Health Annual Report) it was stated that 'Drugs of this group have the advantage of being non-toxic, addiction to them is rare and there are no serious ill effects; they may, therefore, be given to out-patients without due risk.' Eventually Kiloh and Brandon reported that large numbers of patients in Newcastle upon Tyne had become dependent on this drug and had difficulty in stopping using it (Kiloh and Brandon 1962). Also in this decade a steadily increasing number of young people started using amphetamines for recreational purposes. These generally took tablets under the name of 'purple hearts' from their colour and shape. They contained amphetamine and barbiturate. Those who desired a greater effect from amphetamines chewed the contents of inhalers (nasal decongestants) which, at that time, contained very large doses of amphetamine. The third change was the report by Philip Connell that large doses of amphetamines could produce a schizophrenic-like reaction. Although only six cases had been reported previously in this country he described a further forty-two cases of amphetamine psychosis. These were generally young people who had chewed up the contents of amphetamine inhalers to produce a feeling of euphoria (Connell 1958).

Hallucinogens

The 1960s was a decade when taking drugs for recreational and other non-medical reasons became much commoner in some groups. Another drug which was first used in this way at that time was LSD (lysergic acid diethylamide) (Bewley 1967). This was an import from the United States where a local guru called Timothy Leary advocated the use of hallucinogenic drugs to 'expand consciousness' using the slogan 'Turn on, Tune in, and Drop out' (Bryan 1980). He took the view of LSD that 'It was powerful medicine, it is magic, and it has got to be treated that way' (Leary 1970). There was a very small use of psilocybin mushrooms to produce the same effects. The advantage of taking hallucinogens this latter way was that it was completely legal (Cooper 1978).

Sedatives

There was also concern about the over-prescribing of sedatives. In the UK there had always been a history of the use of sedatives to treat minor psychological illnesses. The Victorians had used tincture of laudanum which had been superseded by bromides which in their turn were superseded by barbiturates (following the discovery of cases of chronic bromidism when it became possible to test for this). In the 1960s there was greater awareness of the dangers of the barbiturates. It had been shown very clearly that they could produce severe physical dependence (Isbell 1950). As well as this there was concern about a steady increase in the numbers of people taking overdoses of barbiturates. Though this was sometimes with suicidal intent it was very much more commonly done to attain a temporary respite from the ills and pains of everyday life. For this reason there was a change in the patterns of prescribing sedative drugs. The barbiturates were replaced by benzodiazepines which were much safer when taken for overdose purposes. At that time it was not realised not only that the benzodiazapines were potentially addictive, but also that they could cause dependence when taken in therapeutic doses. They were believed to be very safe hypnotics (Pollitt 1973). The First Report of the Interdepartmental Committee (Ministry of Health 1961) noted that the total quantity of barbiturates prescribed annually in England and Wales had doubled between 1951 and 1959.

Volatile solvents

The final misuse of sedative drugs that was first seen in this decade was the inhalation of volatile solvents. Up to this time the only known problem was found among anaesthetists, who inhaled and at times became addicted to anaesthetic gases. Concern over the death of a child caused by an anaesthetist who sniffed gases led to the Brain Committee being asked to report on this problem among anaesthetists which they did in their Interim Report (Ministry of Health 1959). The new problem was found among much younger people who inhaled different types of solvents to obtain a short-lived feeling of euphoria. The substances varied from the contents of cigarette lighters to airplane glue from model kits, aerosols and other volatile household substances; when inhaled they produced effects similar to alcohol and sometimes hallucinations (Watson 1975).

Responses to changes

One of the effects of the beginnings of a more widespread use of drugs, by young people chiefly, was that there was a great increase in concern about the problems. Newspaper articles on the subject increased. The police were goaded into action. Even Mick Jagger, the then youthful popular singer, was involved. He was arrested for possession of amphetamines and remanded in prison (by the bizarre judge Michael Argyll) where he had a compulsory (regulations) hair cut. Society's over-concern was well expressed in this ridiculous incident described by William Rees Mogg in an editorial as 'Breaking a butterfly upon a wheel' (*The Times* 1967). The response of the young was not unexpected. When later the Beatles were awarded MBEs it was believed, though it is probably an apocryphal story, that they had 'smoked pot' in the men's lavatories in Buckingham Palace on their way to collect their MBEs. As well as smoking cigarettes (generally) drinking alcohol (Ringo Starr excessively: later to become an alcoholic) they were believed to be exponents of hallucinogens – the initials of 'Lucy in the Sky with Diamonds' being the initials of LSD.

There were other, more measured, responses than the temporary gaoling of Jagger on remand. The second Brain Report led the Department of Health to implement its findings. The then Chief Medical Officer Sir George Godber brought about the changes that had been recommended. There was some difficulty with the London teaching hospitals initially, as they did not wish to have anything to do with drug addicts and were unwilling to take on this burden from observation wards and mental hospitals. It was pointed out to them, that their staff were the finest brains in the country and, if they could not deal with this problem, then who could? They did not disagree with this, pointing out that they would be very happy to take this responsibility if only they had the resources. Sir George Godber then played his trump card, 'You can have any money you need from our special contingency fund.' Having been hoisted with their own petard they all set up the necessary centres. (Generally in the most remote part of their subsidiary hospital units.) Sir George of course had the last laugh. The following year when they all said, 'Where is the special money for drug services?,' the Department of Health pointed to their annual block grant and said, 'Right there, bang in the middle of it.' Another response was the setting up of the Institute for the Study of Drug Dependence in 1968 by Frank Logan (with Sir Harry Greenfield, Dick Joyce and Thomas Bewley). Its aims were to provide unbiased accurate information about drug dependence on the basis of its proposed library and information service.

This was much needed as there were no reliable sources of information. At the same time, responding to the needs of homeless young people sleeping rough in the centre of London, many of whom had problems with drugs, the Revd Ken Leech started Centrepoint.

Summary and conclusion

The decade of the 1960s saw a sea change in the drug scene in England. For the very first time some addicts were found to be able to abandon their addiction. The number of doctors who smoked began to decrease leading to a change from two-thirds being smokers to only about one-tenth eventually (Doll and Hill 1964). There was a general increase in consumption of most other drugs. With relative falls in the price of alcohol, the amounts consumed per capita continued to rise and the associated harms also rose. Dependence on prescribed drugs remained relatively unchanged, though dependence on barbiturates was being steadily replaced by dependence on benzodiazepines. The change that caused the greatest concern at that time was the start of the use of illicitly obtained drugs initially for social, recreational and hedonistic purposes. In some cases this led to dependent use. The illnesses associated with all these led to a rethinking of the best medical responses to addiction problems. This led to the setting up of specialised centres for treatment whose main functions were to think and teach. An important development at the time was the realisation that it was not always possible to 'cure' addiction and that there would be many chronic long-term problems in the future. This awareness led to 'Harm reduction' strategies such as advising addicts about how to clean and sterilise syringes and teaching about the dangers of sharing injecting equipment. The development of syringe exchange schemes was started. Drug addiction was believed to be a new problem. Dependence on the socially acceptable drugs had not been recognised to be an identical one. This was the decade when clearer thinking about addiction began to emerge.

References

Bewley, T. H. (1964) Heroin and Cocaine Addiction. *Lancet*, 1: 939.

Bewley, T. H. (1965a) Heroin and Cocaine Addiction. *Lancet*, 2: 808–810.

Bewley, T. H. (1965b) Heroin Addiction in the UK (1954–1964). *British Medical Journal*, 2: 1284–1286.

Bewley, T. H. (1967) Adverse Reaction from the Illicit Use of Lysergide. *British Medical Journal*, 3: 28–30.

Bewley, T. H. (1969a) Drug Dependence in the USA. *Bulletin on Narcotics*, 2: 13–30.

Bewley, T. H. (1969b) The Cannabis Problem in the United Kingdom. *Journal of the American Pharmaceutical Association*, NS 9, 12 December: 613–614.

Bewley, T. H. (1975) Evaluation of Addiction Treatment in England. In *Drug Dependence Treatment and Treatment Evaluation*, eds Bostrom, H., Larsson, T. and Ljungstedt, Stockholm, Sweden, N. Almquist & Wiksell, pp. 287–290.

Bewley, T. H., Ben-Arie, O. and James, I. P. (1968a) Morbidity and Mortality from Heroin Dependence: Survey of Heroin Addicts known to Home Office. *British Medical Journal*, 1: 725–728.

Bewley, T. H. and Ben-Arie, O. (1968b) Morbidity and Mortality from Heroin Dependence: Study of 100 Consecutive Inpatients. *British Medical Journal*, 1: 729–730.

Bewley, T. H., Ben-Arie, O. and Marks, V. (1968c) Morbidity and Mortality from Heroin Dependence: Relation of Hepatitis to Self-injection Techniques. *British Medical Journal*, 1: 730–732.

Bewley, T. H., James, I. P., Le Fevre, Maddox, P. and Mahon, T. (1972) Maintenance Treatment of Narcotic Addicts (Not British nor a System, but Working Now). *International Journal of the Addictions*, 7: 597–611.

Brain, R. (1961) The Report of the Interdepartmental Committee on Drug Addiction. *British Journal of Addiction*, 57: 81–103.

Brewers and Licensed Retailers (1980) *Statistical Handbook*. London, Brewers and Licensed Retailers Publications.

Brown, L. P. (1915) Enforcement of the Tennessee Anti-Narcotics Law, *American Journal of Public Health*, 5: 323–333.

Bryan, J. (1980) *Whatever Happened to Timothy Leary?* San Francisco, USA, Renaissance Press, p. 299.

Connell, P. H. (1958) *Amphetamine Psychosis*. Oxford, Oxford University Press.

Cooper, R. (1978) *A Guide to British Psilocybin Mushrooms*. London, Hassle Free Press.

Dole, V. P. and Nyswander, M. E. (1967) Heroin Addiction – A Metabolic Disease. *Archives of Internal Medicine*, (120): 19–24.

Doll, R. and Hill, A. B. (1964) Mortality in Relation to Smoking: 10 Year Observations of British Doctors. *British Medical Journal*, 1399–1410, 1460–1467.

Frankau, Lady I. M. (1961) Treatment of Heroin and Cocaine Addiction. *Nursing Times*, June, 737–738.

Frankau, Lady I. M. (1964) Treatment in England of Canadian Patients Addicted to Narcotic Drugs. *Canadian Medical Association Journal*, 90, 421–424.

Home Office Cannabis Report by the Advisory Committee on Drug Dependence (1968) (The Wootton Report). London, HMSO.

Isbell, H. (1950) Addiction to Barbiturates and the Barbiturate Abstinence Syndrome. *Archives of Internal Medicine*, (2): 355–397.

Kiloh, L. G. and Brandon, S. (1962) Habituation and Addiction to Amphetamines. *British Medical Journal*, 2: 40–43.

Leary, T. (1970) The Dealer is the New Robin Hood. *International Times*, May, p. 20.

Ministry of Health (1954) Annual Report. London, HMSO, ii, 109.

Ministry of Health (1959) Drug Addiction. Interim Report of the Interdepartmental Committee. London, HMSO.

Ministry of Health (1961) Drug Addiction. Report of the Interdepartmental Committee. London, HMSO.

Ministry of Health (1965) Drug Addiction. Second Report of the Interdepartmental Committee. London, HMSO.

Pollitt, J. D. (1973) The Use of Hypnotics. *Journal of the Royal College of General Practitioners*, 23 (Suppl. 2), 33.

The Times (London), 1967, 1 July 1967 (editorial).

The Times (London), 1967, 24 August 1967, p. 5.

Watson, J. M. (1975) A Study of Solvent Sniffing in Lanarkshire, 1973–1974. *Health Bulletin*, 33 (4): 1–3.

Chapter 5

Crawley New Town

Case study of a local heroin epidemic in the 1960s

N. H. (Raj) Rathod

In the 1960s two notable developments occurred in the field of use of illicit drugs, especially of heroin, in the United Kingdom: (1) an unexpected and unprecedented rise in the numbers using them; and (2) the establishment of provisions both for the treatment of drug addicts and for monitoring the extent of the problem. Up until the early 1960s the observations of the 'Rolleston Committee' (see Chapter 2, this volume) made in 1926 still applied – i.e. that 'addiction to heroin was rare' and was mostly confined to urban areas. However, the numbers of heroin addicts in the UK rose from 62 in 1958 to 1,349 in 1967 (see Chapters 3 and 4, this volume). This upward trend has continued. Until the late 1960s it was believed, as Rolleston had observed, that the problem of addiction was confined to major cities. This would explain the concentration of the special treatment facilities introduced in 1968 in metropolitan cities such as London.

What follows is a sequential account of the epidemiological investigations into the use of heroin in one of the New Towns, Crawley, in the latter half of the 1960s, and supplements the already-published reports. At this point a brief description of the town and the current operating psychiatric services (which carried out the various studies) may be useful.

The town

Crawley New Town is located outside London, but within easy reach of the capital and the popular holiday resorts in the south-east of England. It was one of a number of towns developed to relieve pressure of accommodation in London in the postwar period (Carter, 1974).

Its population grew from 10,000 in 1951 to 64,000 in 1966. It had a young population – the average age of the residents was 30 years, compared with 35 years nationally. The average family consisted of between 3 and 4 people. Forty-five per cent of the residents were under 25 years of age. Seventy-five per cent of the residents were young 'immigrants' from London, having moved there as part of the relocation in the years following the Second

World War, and 90 per cent of the heroin users in Crawley at that time were born in London.

The residential areas were organised into ten self-contained neighbourhoods with easy access to one another and with good shopping, schools and recreational facilities. Employment was not difficult to find. It centred around new engineering firms which needed skilled labour and the expanding Gatwick international airport nearby. Indeed, the local population could not always meet the demands of the labour market. The town's main attractions were good employment prospects, low-cost housing with amenities on hand, a new hospital and good schools, recreational facilities and easy access to holiday resorts.

Local psychiatric services were centred around the newly opened St Christopher's Day Hospital situated in Horsham, a market town eight miles south of Crawley. Emphasis was on the development of services centred in the community, which would provide an alternative to in-patient services as far as was feasible.

The in-patient services were based at Graylingwell hospital in Chichester, some 40 miles distant from Crawley. This obviously helped the objectives of the local psychiatric services as it promoted development of close liaison with various local helping agencies. Two newly-appointed consultants (N. H. Rathod and R. de Alarcon) and a trainee psychiatrist were in charge of developing local services for a population of over 130,000 covering Crawley, Horsham and the surrounding rural areas. Circumstances favoured autonomy and the development of initiatives.

First signs of heroin

Until 1966 there was no reason to suspect heroin abuse of any magnitude in Crawley. However, this assumption was soon proved wrong. In March/April 1967 two boys aged 17 and 19 were referred for treatment of heroin addiction. They claimed that they had been injecting heroin for months and that there were many others like them in the town. This came as a surprise and was hard to believe. It prompted us to question more closely two other teenagers whom we had treated in the latter half of 1966 for oral amphetamine abuse. We were unpleasantly surprised to discover that they too had used heroin regularly before admission. It was obvious we had missed this important clinical detail – a classic example of 'no suspicion, no investigation'.

These events alerted us to the possibility of a sizeable public health and clinical problem in our midst which needed investigating. The need was reinforced by an increasing number of referrals, and approaches by parents, teachers and others from Crawley for advice on how to detect heroin use and what to do about it. From our clinical standpoint, early intervention required early diagnosis.

The situation presented us with a unique opportunity and a challenge to investigate heroin use locally. The presentation that follows is divided into three parts:

1   the first part deals with the search for clues in the diagnosis of heroin use and identifying users;
2   the second part deals with the estimation of the size of the problem, methods of spread of use, and the monitoring of trends over time; and
3   the third part deals with following individuals' patterns of use and outcome *vis-à-vis* use of heroin over a period of years.

The diagnostic challenge

We found the text books of little practical value. Signs such as nausea, respiratory depression, pupillary size and such were difficult to elicit in practice. Reliance on patients' accounts could be equally misleading. Moreover, our experience in this field was extremely limited, which further hampered us.

We were told repeatedly by our patients that they had little difficulty in recognising a 'junkie' in the streets, in recognising who was 'under the influence' or 'stoned', and who was experiencing withdrawal or a 'comedown'. These assertions were difficult to ignore. We turned to these experiential 'experts' for guidance and initiated an exercise to investigate the authenticity of their claims. We hoped to identify reliable and useful pointers or signs and symptoms which could be of use to us as well as to others. As a pilot study, twelve patients and twelve parents participated individually in drawing up a list of clues which they thought were most likely to identify states of being 'stoned' or a 'comedown'. Parents were prompted to list any recent changes in appearance, demeanour or behaviour of their offspring which they found difficult to understand or which made them suspect drug use. Each participant did the exercise independently. The result was 38 items with varying degrees of concordance between the two groups. A month later, a group of 20 patients and parents were asked to rate each of these 38 items, according to their relevance in detecting use of heroin – as 'Yes', 'No', or 'Do not know'. As in the initial exercise, the responses of patients were far more accurate, both for the signs of people being under the influence of drugs and for states of withdrawal. On the other hand, the parents' observations on behaviour, appearance, etc. were much more to the point. The consistency between the responses for both groups on each of these occasions could not be ignored. Later on, a member of the staff, not directly involved with the patient, was invited to observe a patient in an interview situation and to use the 38 items in this inventory to diagnose whether the patient was under the influence of heroin or was withdrawing (we knew of the approximate time of the patient's last injection). On occasion, a non-drug-user patient would substitute a heroin patient in the interview. Out of a total of 29 test occasions, wrong diagnosis was made on only two. To find a pharmacological basis for many of the signs named by the patients was reassuring. We had gained some useful guidelines for diagnosis of heroin use during different phases of the pharmacological effects. For example, the behaviour of rubbing of the eyes and the peri-oral areas finds its likely explanation in the release of histamine by opioids. Similarly, parental reports of recent repeated attacks of 'flu-like' symptoms were in reality evidence of minor withdrawal phenomena. We used these pointers a good deal in our work and used them in public talks. Interestingly the patients' listings displayed a remarkable lack of awareness on their part of their behaviour and general demeanour while they were under the influence or withdrawing, i.e. they displayed a lack of insight (Rathod et al., 1967).

Although the diagnostic indicators proved useful to us, we could not confirm their relative specificity because they have neither been challenged nor confirmed in any other sample since this study. The items were particularly useful in detecting use in the early stages of heroin use and by implication in assisting non-medical people in detection in the early stages – which we considered important, since we believed that earlier detection would be likely to be associated with early intervention and a better outcome.

Involvements of patients and parents in a 'hands-on' exercise revealed the potential of both groups in making a valuable contribution to the understanding of the manifestations of heroin use. It became clear that the varied information could well be useful in helping the users as well as the observers in bridging the gap of misunderstanding and confusion. It is probable that this exercise raised the confidence of most participants as having something positive to contribute towards helping drug users.

Estimating extent of use and mode of spread

The ideal method of identifying the maximum numbers would have been to use a field survey and to interview those in the 'at risk' group. However, such an exercise was beyond the scope of a busy general psychiatric service such as ours, leaving aside the question of the reliability of information received.

Our traditional sources of information had been referrals from GPs and from the courts. Sole reliance on these would grossly underestimate the extent of the problem, as non-referrals far exceed referrals. Use of heroin was, and still is, regarded as something deviant and a desire to avoid disclosure is inevitable and indeed understandable. Also the users in the early stage experience few if any problems, as the pleasant immediate experiences ('the buzz' or 'the kick') far outweigh the unpleasant ones.

We decided to seek information from the sources more likely to come across users – Police and Probation services, and the patients themselves. We also used two indirect methods, namely a survey within the local casualty department and a local survey of the incidence of jaundice.

Police and Probation services

Our efforts to form close links with local agencies proved useful. Each nominated a senior officer who acted as our link person. One of us acted as a liaison man from our team and had regular meetings with the officers and received information on anyone who was suspected, searched, arrested or convicted of using drugs, especially heroin, or admitted to using heroin (e.g. to a probation officer). In between such meetings, individual officers also gave information. All information was given and treated in confidence. They respected our inability to divulge any information about a patient.

Surveys of medical complications

These were frequent amongst our patients, jaundice being one and overdoses being another. Our experience was not unique, as others also had noticed outbreaks of hepatitis among heroin addicts (e.g. Bewley, 1965). Inspired by Jellinek's use of frequency of cirrhosis of the liver to estimate the extent of alcoholism, and Sherlock's dictum that 'any patient developing jaundice within six months of any procedure involving puncture of the skin must be assumed to have contracted serum jaundice unless proven otherwise', we surveyed all general practices in Crawley and recorded the names of all those aged between 15 and 25 who had jaundice during 1966 and 1967. We searched the records of the local casualty department for all cases of overdose with stimulants and/or hypnotics which had involved young people between the ages of 15 and 25 during the whole of 1966 and 1967. With both the jaundice survey and the overdose survey, all the cases turned out to be under the age of 21 years and all were Crawley residents.

Direct information from patients

We had a strong feeling that our patients knew a good deal about who was involved locally with drug use and about other aspects of the lives of their associates. The main problem was their reluctance to divulge any information because they thought that this might get the friend into trouble, and that it would be tantamount to 'grassing'. Repeated reassurance about confidentiality was needed and we adhered to it strictly. Sometimes we resorted to unorthodox methods, such as one of us recording the information in Hindi (an Indian language) which no one else in the service could read at that time. Over time, mutual confidence grew and patients contributed valuable information – both of a personal nature and relating to drug habits. This information was often qualitatively rich, as their associations went back to school days as well as the neighbourhood experiences.

Patients were encouraged to provide the names of the users they knew, to discuss who had initiated them (who gave them their first 'fix') and where and when this took place and those whom they themselves initiated, as well as any other information of relevance.

Cumulative case register

In this way, a cumulative case register was started. Information from all the screening methods was entered, continuously updated and cross-checked. Each patient had his own data sheet (referred to as 'the diary'). Entries included the usual basic demographic data, main points on drug use, etc. In addition the first screening method to name or identify the patient, date of the information, points on initiation, etc. were enquired into and entered as a matter of routine. The first screening method to name a user was credited as the identifying screening method. The quality and quantity of information obviously varied but only in a minority of cases was it scant.

Heroin use was classified as: (A) *Confirmed* if the patient was under treatment for heroin use, convicted for possession, or admitted to use of heroin to the police or probation officers; (B) *Probable* if named by only two sources other than those already themselves listed as 'Confirmed'; and (C) *Suspected* if named by only one source other than those listed themselves in the 'Confirmed' category.

Ninety-eight names were entered in the cumulative register between 1 May and 31 December 1967. Of these, 50 were confirmed, 5 were probable and 37 were suspects. Viewed according to the first source of information, eight confirmed cases were attributed to GP referrals and the remaining 42 to the other identification methods. By the end of the survey 15 more cases were referred by GPs and we had 31 patients under our care. The screening methods which proved most rewarding were the patients themselves and the jaundice survey. Of the 46 people named by patients, 17 were 'confirmed' (and more were confirmed later). The jaundice survey revealed 20 names, of whom 8 were confirmed. The casualty overdose survey revealed 8 people being treated for amphetamine overdose, of whom 4 were confirmed as heroin users. Police and probation services named 9, of whom 8 were confirmed (4 had been convicted). All the patients were under the age of 21 years, Crawley residents, and 90 per cent were male. Based on our definition of a case, and bearing in mind that not all the cases might have been identified, the prevalence rate for both sexes for the age group 15 to 20 (total population 5,880), and expressed as rate per 1000 was 8.50 for confirmed and 0.85 for probable cases. The rates for males only was higher at 14.75 for confirmed and 1.64 for probable cases.

Of the 31 cases seen by us, all were injecting the drug intravenously. Eight patients claimed to be injecting no more than twice a week and to have started using heroin in the last six months. The rest claimed to be using heroin more than three days a week and nine of them for 18 months (or more). For further details see de Alarcon and Rathod (1968).

During this survey we learnt that most of the spread occurred in an atmosphere of convivial sharing, an experienced user initiating a friend and 'training' the initiate how to inject – thus a habit was passed from person to person. Sharing often included preparation of the 'fix' and sharing equipment, and buying supplies for each other. Sharing was restricted to people well known and trusted. In other words sharing occurred between people who felt close to each other. Patients often described them as belonging to an 'inner circle' – usually made up of four to six. Closeness of association determined its boundaries. This description is analogous to the spread of an infection from person to person by personal contact and reminds one of the observation by Morris (1957) that, 'There are many interesting analogies between the dynamics of infectious disease and that of mental illness: from the dancing mania of the Middle Ages to the epidemic of Benzedrine addiction.' Postulation of spread by personal transmission resulted in information on initiation thereafter being sought as a routine part of our clinical history taking. Cross-checking the information from the initiator and the initiate resulted in data which supported the hypothesis of transmission from person to person.

By September 1968 we had seen 51 patients, who were initiated during or prior to the end of 1967. All were under 20 years of age, and residents of Crawley; 42 had named their initiator and gave approximate date of initiation, and 8 provided information only on approximate date of initiation. As a result of this mapping, two users were identified as the source of the entire spread. Both were residents of Crawley who had been initiated in two coastal towns in the south and prior to 1965. From these saplings, as it were, two sizeable trees grew rapidly. Twenty-four were initiated in 1966, and twenty-six in 1967. Thus it was the Crawley residents who were responsible for starting, and continuing, the spread of this 'epidemic'. The spread has been reported elsewhere (de Alarcon, 1969), and is figuratively shown in Figure 5.1.

Characteristics of the heroin users

There was little that was distinctive about the group as a whole and there was nothing definitive that could be used to identify a person at risk. However, a minority had evidence of exposure to disturbing emotional experiences within their families and signs of delinquency before the age of 15 and before their use of any illicit drugs. In other words, there were indications of maladjustment predating their drug use. Evidence showing that these features were not shared by others of similar age came from two different studies from Crawley. In a pilot study, 30 male heroin patients (surnames starting with letters A to I) were compared with 27 general psychiatric patients with no evidence of drug use – all from Crawley and of similar age. Information was gathered on the parents and families from GPs' notes, from the Child Guidance Clinic and from Probation Officers. In 20 of the

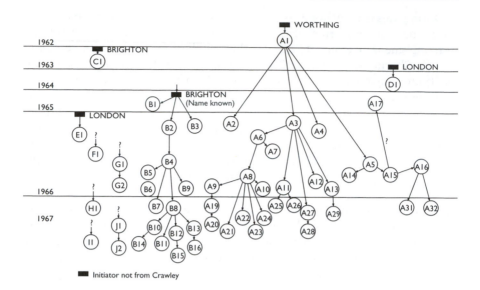

Figure 5.1 The spread from the Crawley epidemic
Source: *Bulletin on Narcotics*, vol. XXI, no. 3: 18.

30 heroin patients there was history of parental divorce or separation, and/ or sustained problems in the parents associated with alcohol, hypnotics or stimulants use. Nine of the general psychiatric patients had a history of parental break-up of marriage only. Although a third in each group had received help from the Child Guidance Clinic, nine of the heroin patients had a diagnosis of conduct disorders as opposed to only one in the general group. In addition, half of the heroin patients had a proven history of delinquency before the use of drugs, as compared to none in the general psychiatric group (Rathod, 1972). Another piece of evidence came from a later study. At the time of the heroin 'epidemic' in Crawley, the Home Office had started a study on juvenile delinquents in Crawley – called the Crawley Juvenile (CJ) Project. It compared a group of delinquents with a matched control group from Crawley on various parameters including family backgrounds and, of course, delinquency. This gave us the opportunity to compare our heroin users with the non-drug-using delinquents and the non-delinquents cohort (controls) from the CJ Project who acted as controls. As expected, the heroin group matched well with the other two groups – after all, they had all been reared in a similar general environment. The number of males involved in each group was 66 in the heroin group, 89 in the non-drug-using delinquents group, and 77 in the control group. Using referral to a Child Guidance Clinic as a measure of maladjustment, no one in the control group,

13 per cent amongst the delinquent group and 23 per cent in the heroin group were referred. The percentage of those in the heroin group who were convicted of an offence before their first admitted misuse of drugs was twice as high as expected – 35 per cent compared with 15 per cent (Mott and Rathod, 1976). However, it was evident that a history of delinquency on its own was not a sufficient condition for becoming a heroin user.

Of special interest may be those in this group who displayed social deviancy at an early age and may thus be more likely to perpetuate that pattern and thus be more vulnerable to long-term use of narcotics or other drugs deemed as illegal by society. In a study in which 86 of the local heroin users were followed for up to six years, it was found that social maladjustment prior to use of illegal drugs and continued use of drugs by injection were closely associated (Rathod, 1977).

Studying the extent of spread of heroin and its nature

The screening methods in combination proved a reliable source of data and their validity was strengthened through cross-checking procedures. Patients' contributions exceeded our expectations. As we provided no prescribed maintenance treatment, they had little to gain from misleading us. Their information was more often confirmed than contradicted by events. Their potential contribution to research in various aspects of drug use in a community is generally overlooked and undervalued.

Another tool little used in research is morbidity associated with drug use as an indicator of drug use in a community. Study of levels of morbidity vary greatly according to the condition under study and the geographical area and time. Common occurrence and easy accessibility of data are major advantages and may override the disadvantage of non-specificity. While not every overdose implies use of illicit drugs, use of illicit drugs is a major contributor to overdoses. Our own experience as well as that of others (Ghodse, 1977) indicates that data on overdoses can be used to gauge the extent of use of a particular drug and its related morbidity in the community. Furthermore, the changing nature of overdoses can reflect the changing preferences. Similarly, although serum hepatitis only identifies the method of administration of a drug (i.e. by injection) and not the drug itself, changes in the frequency with which it occurs can serve as an indicator of the prevalence of intravenous drug use and/or the effectiveness or otherwise of attempts at introducing better hygiene in self-administration of drugs. Reduction in frequency of overdoses as well as hepatitis may, on another level, reflect the reduced morbidity associated with a change to a less risky route of taking a drug, e.g. from injecting to smoking. Attention to such a possibility has been drawn in relation to smoking heroin (Strang et al., 1992) but no proper study to test this possibility has yet been undertaken. Mortality is another complication that may prove useful and relatively easy to track and to study.

Was the Crawley experience unique?

This is a difficult question to answer because of absence of similar enquiries in another New Town at that time. A more useful question may be: 'Does the Crawley experience indicate that in the late 1960s young people in their late teens became a population at risk of using potent narcotics (heroin) or stimulants (methedrine)?' The answer is likely to be 'yes' as shown by Home Office data on narcotics in the late 1960s. Crawley or any similar town with a large concentration of young people did provide the most suitable host for such an epidemic and similar problems were also reported from other towns or cities (Kosviner *et al.*, 1968).

The reported prevalence rates are probably a true reflection of the prevailing situation. This assumption is based on two factors. A wide variety of screening methods was used, constantly cross-checked and information updated. Second, ours was the only psychiatric service available to users and no outside facility was yet accessible, as the special treatment units were not yet operational.

Our analogy of an epidemic spread by contagion may revive memories of the sterile debate about the 'medical model' where a behaviour (in this case taking drugs) and its consequences are 'medicalised'. The argument is academic because what matters is the phenomenon and not the label. The most striking feature about the spread was that it was sudden and unforeseen, started and sustained by residents of the town and contained within the community. Also of interest is the fact that to the best of our knowledge, everyone used the intravenous route. Also we neither saw nor knew of any case in 1967–1968 in the town of Horsham just eight miles south of Crawley or other places we served nearby. At that time there was no evidence of 'pushers' from outside. All these facts tempt one to postulate that it was primarily a shared social experience on a major scale and without evidence of any consideration for the possible consequences. In this sense it was a unique occurrence. We have already postulated as to what made Crawley so vulnerable a host. If this were correct the epidemic should prove to be self-limiting provided no outside factors intervened. The discussion on the trends that followed supports that paradigm.

Monitoring trends after the original 'epidemic'

Trends were properly monitored only until October 1970. The same screening methods as before were used. By October 1970 there were 139 names on the register – 102 of these were 'Confirmed' cases, 4 'Probable' and 33 'Suspects'. Of the Confirmed, 85 were male; the ratio of M:F remaining the same, i.e. 5 to 1. Ninety-one patients were seen and diagnosed as Confirmed.

So far 17 girls were diagnosed as Confirmed, with none in the Probable category and 14 in the Suspected group. Interestingly, the majority of the

Confirmed girls were identified by medical sources or by police, i.e. 13 out of 17 (6 per cent as opposed to 47 per cent of the boys). The overdose survey identified none and the users themselves named only a handful extra. Prevalence rates for the whole group declined every year from 8.2 per 1000 in 1967 to 3.6 in 1970. However, the rate for 20 to 24 years age group showed a slight increase from 3.6 in 1967 to 4.3 in 1970. Incidence rates were calculated on the basis of the recorded year of initiation. The rates for those in the initiation age group 14 to 19 declined every year from 6.5 in 1967 to 0.82 in 1970.

Learning lessons from the Crawley experience

Consistent decline in the prevalence and incidence of heroin use in Crawley may be taken as supporting the hypothesis that the spread of heroin in Crawley was primarily the result of convivial sharing between old acquaintances and should therefore be self-limiting. However, it could be argued that a period as short as three years (1967 to 1970) is not sufficient to forecast trends. The rise in prevalence rates among the 20 to 24 years age group suggests that a nucleus of long-term users was developing. These people could act both as active cases as well as carriers of the drug-using behaviour to new initiates. The girls as a group show some puzzling features. Contrary to the usual expectation, none of them had a history or evidence of overdose. They were mostly successful in keeping their drug-taking behaviour secret. It is difficult to explain why the majority were identified by doctors and the police rather than by other sources, as was the case with boys.

Circumstances beyond our control resulted in significant reduction, in the latter half of 1968, in the senior and junior staff interested in the work with drug users. Shortage of staff and the changed ambience did affect all aspects of the work adversely. This must have blunted the screening methods and recording of data. That is one major reason why the study in trends was, regrettably, not pursued. Studies in trends are a very good guide to the effectiveness or otherwise of preventive and therapeutic measures. They also reflect how effective are the measures aimed at controlling demand and supply.

Looking back 30 years later

Looking back, I think that Richard de Alarcon and I embarked on a journey into the unknown when undertaking this work, but we found it an exciting and rewarding one. The study had its origin in our shared approach to clinical research, which was never to dismiss unexpected clinical incidents without attempting to test their veracity and clinical implications. Being inexperienced in detecting or managing 'narcotic addiction', we were caught unawares when we independently encountered two heroin injectors, in a small provincial town like Crawley, and even more surprised at the patients' claim that there were many more. Several exciting exercises followed – discovering the signs and symptoms from the people experiencing them, using medical complications as screening tools, establishing the convivial channels of the spread of initiating people, and using community helping agencies. We learned not to underestimate the value of the patient as a research tool, and the ease with which the drug-incepting behaviour can spread.

Further follow-up of this cohort is planned to find out what has happened to them, and this will further advance our understanding of the critical points and pathways of the local spread of heroin misuse, and its relationship to the unfolding of associated harms.

References

Bewley, T. H. (1965). Heroin and cocaine addiction. *Lancet*, 808–10.

Carter, G. (1974). Town planning in Crawley. Crawley Urban District Council.

De Alarcon, R. (1969). The spread of heroin abuse in a community. *UN Bulletin of Narcotics*, 21: 17–22.

De Alarcon, R. and Rathod, N. H. (1968). Prevalence and early detection of heroin abuse. *British Medical Journal*, 2: 549–53.

Ghodse, A. H. (1977). Drug dependent individuals dealt with by London Casualty Departments. *British Journal of Psychiatry*, 131: 273–80.

Jellinek, E. M. (1960). *The Disease Concept of Alcoholism*. New Haven: Hillhouse Press.

Kosviner, A., Mitcheson, M., Myers, K., Ogborne, A., Stimson, G. V., Zacune, J. and Edwards, G. (1968). Heroin use in a provincial town. *Lancet*, I: 1189–92.

Morris, T. N. (1957). *Uses of Epidemiology*. E. & S. Livingston Ltd.

Mott, J. and Rathod, N. H. (1976). Heroin misuse and delinquency in a new town. *British Journal of Psychiatry*, 128: 428–35.

Rathod, N. H. (1972). The use of heroin and methadone by injection in a new town: progress report. *British Journal of Addiction*, 67: 113–22.

Rathod, N. H. (1977). Follow-up study of injectors in a provincial town. *Drug and Alcohol Dependence*, 2: 1–21.

Rathod, N. H., de Alarcon, R. and Thomson, I. G. (1967). Signs of heroin usage detected by drug users and their parents. *Lancet*, 2: 1411–14.

Strang, J., Des Jarlais, D., Griffiths, P. and Gossop, M. (1992). The study of transitions in the route of drug use: the route from one route to another. *British Journal of Addiction*, 87: 473–83.

Chapter 6

Intravenous and oral street use of barbiturates

The 'epidemic' of the 1970s and early 1980s

Angela Burr

Introduction

This chapter describes the history of the barbiturate misuse 'epidemic' that hit, in particular, London in the 1970s, and outlines its physical, social and symbolic dimensions. It examines the symbolic usage of barbiturates by Punks and Skinheads, the Piccadilly drug scene, the club-going scene and 'Barb Freaks'. It also describes the impact the epidemic had on service provision, including the opening of City Roads, the crisis intervention centre. It points as well to the policy lessons that need to be learnt from the epidemic.

The ability of barbiturates to calm and produce drowsiness or sleep led to them being viewed as a miracle drug for the treatment of sleep and anxiety problems when they were first introduced early in the twentieth century. But evidence gradually began to appear indicating that they have a high potential for abuse, for overdosing and physical dependence and that they can be lethal in overdose. Even so, until the 1980s, millions of barbiturates were medically prescribed. In 1971 alone, English doctors wrote out 12.9 million prescriptions for barbiturates. Teff (1975: 199) estimated that 100,000 people were dependent on them in 1966.

Their lethal nature became particularly apparent in Britain in the 1970s and early 1980s, when their illicit street non-medical use developed into a serious problem in the London drug scene. A barbiturate misuse 'epidemic' occurred, particularly amongst the injecting population. Similar use was also reported in Edinburgh (Forrest and Tarala 1973) and in northern cities, such as the Manchester and Bradford club scenes (Tyler 1988).

An injecting barbiturate problem develops

By the late 1960s, injectors had discovered that barbiturates could be crushed and injected and an injecting subculture had developed in London. Referred to as 'barbs', 'downers' or 'sleepers', barbiturates such as Tuinal (quinalbarbitone and amylobarbitone), Nembutal (pentobarbitone sodium), Amytal (amylobarbitone) and Seconal (quinalbarbitone sodium) became easily available and extensively used – especially within the West End Picca-dilly pharmaceutical illicit drug market and subculture, the heart of the London drug scene, which had grown up during the 1960s and supplied much of the capital's black market in pharmaceutical drugs. The barbiturate black market was fed mainly by the overspill from general practitioners, forged prescriptions and chemist and pharmaceutical warehouse thefts and for a short time after they were set up, from Drug Dependency Units (DDUs).

These barbiturate users have generally been characterised as poly- or multiple substance users. Mitcheson *et al.* (1970, 1971), for example, in a study of 65 primarily heroin users, carried out at three day centres in 1969, found that 62 had used barbiturates, 52 had injected them and 65 per cent had used them for hedonistic purposes. But it was not just opiate addicts who used barbiturates. Many, particularly young people, used a wide variety of substances, including opiates, barbiturates, amphetamines and alcohol. Whilst some remained occasional users and never became dependent on any substance, some did become dependent. In fact, a subculture developed in which barbiturates were the preferred or even the only substance used. This was particularly the case with drug-using Punks and Skinheads who fre-quented the Piccadilly and Kensington Market drug scenes at the beginning of the 1980s (Burr 1984b).

Barbiturates were, at the time, the most dangerous and lethal drug used by substance misusers. People who use them regularly soon become physically tolerant and have to use more and more to get the same effect. Immediate withdrawal can lead to convulsions, delirium, hallucinations, hypothermia, high fever and even coma and death. The withdrawals can be so severe heavy users quickly take more. These effects foster a powerful need to continue taking them and often heavy users become incapable of living without them. Also, with heavy daily use, the margin between tolerance and overdose level rapidly decreases, often resulting in overdose and death. If injected, physical complications can occur such as abscesses and ulcerations. Also arms and legs may become gangrenous if there is accidental injection into the artery, dirty needles are used or dangerous cutting substances added to the capsule.

Heavy barbiturate users, if they stay awake, exhibit symptoms similar to drunkenness. They are unable to think clearly and become confused. As a consequence the risk of fatal overdose is high, particularly as the higher doses needed to get 'stoned' get dangerously close to the fatal overdose level as the user becomes tolerant to the drug and needs higher doses to get the same effect (what the pharmacologist would call 'reduced therapeutic margin'). Often they fall into unconsciousness. Stoned and oblivious to the world, they neglect themselves, their behaviour becomes chaotic and their social life disintegrates. Lacking co-ordination, they are prone to accidents and often fall down and injure themselves. Their lack of emotional control and hostility engendered by supposed insults often leads to their becoming quarrelsome, aggressive and violent.

It was a common daily sight in Piccadilly, for example, during the 1970s and early 1980s, to see dishevelled 'Barb Freaks', as barbiturate users were called, staggering about, lying overdosed on the pavements or public lavatories or sleeping off the effects in doorways or getting into fights and injuring themselves, or with abscesses from injecting or with amputated fingers or a missing limb.

The barbiturate misuse morbidity and mortality rate became massive as is clear from Ghodse *et al.*'s (1998) graph (see Figure 6.1) which shows the proportion of addict deaths per year between 1967 and 1993 which relate to different types of drug. Barbiturates killed more addicts than heroin during the 1970s and were implicated in more than half the addict deaths in 1972, only tailing off towards the end of the 1970s. In fact, the extensive use of barbiturates still continued in Piccadilly between 1979 and 1981 (Burr 1983, 1984b; Tyler 1988: 106–107).

London Casualty Departments, particularly the five central London ones (Ghodse 1976, 1977) became inundated with 'Barb Freaks' needing treatment for overdosing and injuries. In a survey (Ghodse 1977) in August 1975 of 395 drug-dependent individuals dealt with by 62 Greater London Casualty Departments, the majority of whom were seen following an overdose, barbiturates were the drug most frequently used. At the Middlesex Hospital in central London, many unconscious addicts were brought in two or three

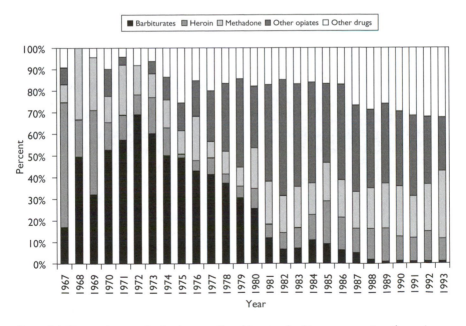

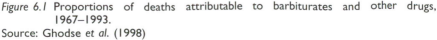

Figure 6.1 Proportions of deaths attributable to barbiturates and other drugs, 1967–1993.
Source: Ghodse *et al.* (1998)

times over a single 24-hour period (Mitchell and Rose 1975: 1489). Their disruptive and aggressive behaviour hindered the Casualty's normal work – similarly the local voluntary agencies such as the Hungerford, CDP and New Horizon, all of whom, by 1975, had felt obliged to close their fixing rooms.

A range of studies, e.g. in Day Centres (Mitcheson 1970, 1971), in Drug Dependence Units (DDUs) (D'Orban 1976; Teggin and Bewley 1979), in Casualties (Ghodse 1976, 1977, 1979; Ghodse and Rawson 1978a; Mitchell and Rose 1975), on the street (Burr 1983, 1984a, 1984b) and from mortality statistics (Stevens 1978; Ghodse *et al.*, 1998), revealed the extent and nature of the problem. SCODA undertook a survey in 1973 of the Central London street agencies which showed that half the number of people seen, about 200, were using barbiturates regularly. Replies to a questionnaire (D'Orban 1976: 65) sent to London DDUs in September 1975 showed that, on average, 37 per cent of patients were using barbiturates and, for 15 per cent of these addicts, it was considered a serious problem.

There were a range of reasons for the barbiturate 'epidemic'. The extensive intravenous abuse of methylamphetamine at the end of the 1960s has often been viewed as the catalyst linking the London pill culture with the injecting subculture. After methylamphetamine was taken off the market in the late 1960s, injectors had to look for other drugs, and barbiturates' injectability made them attractive.

Mitcheson (1994: 184) has also argued that the end of the Vietnam War led to several years of drought in the Golden Triangle which restricted the supply of street heroin. This will have been compounded by the decrease in the availability of injectable heroin due to the DDU's policy of moving away from prescribing injectables in the 1970s (see Chapter 4, Volume II, by Martin Mitcheson). These factors also acted as catalysts to the injecting barbiturate problem, especially in Central London. Certainly addicts used the latter argument to justify a return to prescribing injectables and bigger scripts throughout the 1970s. But other injectable drugs, such as amphetamine sulphate and Ritalin (methylphenidate hydrocol) were available at the time, so the injectability of barbiturates alone does not explain the choice or continued use of barbiturates during the 1970s, particularly as their physical effects were very different from opiates. Nor does their injectability explain their attraction for those who only swallowed them.

The easy availability of supplies of barbiturates, both for dealers and users, played a significant role in their use. So, too, did their cheapness – two capsules of Tuinal, for example, in 1980, cost one pound in Piccadilly. This was a major attraction to many heavy barbiturate users, as they were mostly unemployed and too chaotic and dishevelled to shoplift or do credit card frauds and as a result were unable to finance an expensive methadone or heroin habit. But amphetamines and cannabis were also relatively cheap, as was alcohol (e.g. Special Brew) which could be used to achieve a somewhat similar effect, so cost alone cannot totally account for barbiturate use either, particularly by those who used only occasionally. Barbiturates were also used by prostitutes working in the West End/Piccadilly area and some of the better-off could certainly have afforded, at least some of the time, to use more expensive drugs.

The characterisation of barbiturate users as poly- or multiple drug misusers, however, somewhat misrepresents the situation with regard to reasons for using barbiturates. Some indiscriminately used any drug available, whilst others preferred amphetamines and used barbiturates to counteract the agitation induced by their stimulating effects or they preferred barbiturates and used amphetamines to negate the latter's soporific qualities. Some heroin or methadone users only used them when no other drug was available. But, for others, both occasional and heavy users, barbiturates, particularly Tuinal, was their drug of preference. This was especially the case with drug-using Punks and Skinheads towards the end of the 1970s.

The lifestyle and symbolic dimension of barbiturate misuse

This preference for barbiturates needs to be understood and was explored in Burr (1984b) (the following section is a summary of this analysis). It is necessary to explore the role that the human body plays in contemporary Western society. Also how drugs fit in with the beliefs, values, concerns and lifestyles of youth and addict subcultures and their symbolic usage of drugs.

The human body is a universal medium for basic human perception and symbolic interaction everywhere. There has been an increase in bodily awareness and bodily symbolism has become all pervasive. Indeed, a 'cult of the body' has developed. A reason for this bodily focus may be found in individuals who, unable to find answers to their problems in the increasingly fragmented and competitive society in which they live, have turned from the constraints and confinement of an unacceptable social environment to themselves and their inner psyches to deal with the problems they face in their daily lives. They have sought freedom and solutions to their problems through the medium of their bodies and bodily symbolism. There is, nowadays, particularly amongst marginal groups, an increasing manipulation, both conscious and unconscious, of the values and symbols assigned to bodily categories as a form of self-expression, self-realisation and social protest.

A variety of social and economic reasons underlie contemporary illicit substance misuse. Drugs and the bodily experiences and behaviour they generate, are another way the body is used for expressing and dealing with social problems. They offer a prime metaphor for symbolic revolt. Because their chemical contents affect the body in a variety of ways, they offer a flexible and wide range of forms of bodily expression, particularly those that can be injected and consequently entail a great deal of bodily ritual.

Punks and Skinheads and the symbolic usage of barbiturates

Hall *et al.* (1976) have interpreted the modern youth subcultures as forms of revolt and systems of problem solving, as reactions against both the parent working-class culture and the dominant hegemony and ideology of the ruling power structure. They view youth movements as providing solutions on the ideological and ritual level, by means of their dress, activities and lifestyle to the problems imposed on them by their working-class position in society, such as alienation and their humdrum existence caused by poor employment prospects and repetitive poorly paid unskilled jobs. But youth movements have turned to 'style' as Hebdige (1979) has referred to this form of social protest, precisely because it is a medium which centres on and is articulated through the body and provides a vehicle for bodily symbolism.

The acuteness of the problems faced by the 40 drug-using Punks and Skinheads interviewed in my study (Burr 1984b) is indicated by their social profiles. They came from highly disrupted family backgrounds, had a high rate of non-drug-related delinquency and a history of unemployment.

Substance-misusing Punks and Skinheads sought answers to their problems in negative and self-destructive ways and by expressing their frustration and despair on the symbolic level. They projected onto their subcultures, both their grim existence, the feeling of alienation and problems faced by working-class youth in general in their daily lives, and their own fundamentally disrupted family and social backgrounds. The beliefs, values, concerns and lifestyles of their subcultures developed an equally disturbed and destructive outlook which may be called 'Ideologies of Despair'.

Their choice of barbiturates was neither random nor accidental. Cannabis, the happy euphoria-inducing 'make love not war' drug of the Hippies, would not have fitted in with the outlook of the Punk or Skinhead subculture. Nor would the amphetamines which fuelled the weekend party scene of 'pillheads' in the early 1960s. Barbiturates became their preferred drug – precisely because of their lethal potential and the aggressive and chaotic behaviour they fostered. This was not an unwanted complication, for it fitted in with their disturbed self-destructive outlooks and epitomised the negative nihilist attitude embodied in their subcultures. Barbiturates offered a particularly meaningful and powerful symbol for articulating their social predicament, their despair with their social lives and their social protest.

Punks

Punks first appeared in 1976. Working-class in ethic, they embodied a total alienation from society and rejection of conventional working-class society. Punks were not accidentally offensive; they explicitly aimed to shock and be offensive and outrage straight society. They personified an 'ideology of inversion'. Everything valued by conventional society was inverted by

Punks and detested. Everything 'society' detested was valued. Punks wore their cultural style on their bodies. They valued outrageous hairstyles, tatty clothing, the wearing of pedal bin liners, swastikas and bondage chains and the piercing of their bodies with crude safety pins. They glorified cockney speech, foul language, vulgarity, spitting in public places, sexual perversity and villainy.

The inherent dangers in using barbiturates – becoming heavily stoned, the staggering about and the dishevelled appearance of users and the blotting out of awareness – fitted in with their subcultural style and provided another ideal medium for expressing their destructive outlook and total rejection of society. As Punks often said when asked why they used barbiturates, 'It's the only fucking way you can get out of the fucking system.' Along with their bondage chains, barbiturates had the appeal of cheapness and identification with the poverty-stricken low-status end of the addict drug scene, which provided another medium for identifying with, and assuming, the stigmata of the lowly and downtrodden with whom Punks identified. They offered, too, a clear contrast to the 'safe' use of tranquillisers which during the 1970s became a symbol and panacea for all of the ills in Western society.

Skinheads

Skinheads first appeared in the 1960s and again in the mid-1970s. They were a symbolic antithesis to Punks, though they had an equally alienated, negative outlook. They focused on positive action and involvement. They strongly identified, albeit in a parodied form, with conventional society and conformed to a version of pre-war working-class values which no longer exists.

This conformity was expressed by a strong commitment to the traditional male machismo role. Fighting to protect what they perceived to be working-class values became a skinhead focal concern. The machismo role and fighting were particularly attractive to unemployed working-class youth. Unable to express their masculinity and unable to achieve status and self-esteem through their jobs, becoming a 'Skinhead' offered them an alternative means of doing so.

However, the machismo role and status, evaluated in terms of fighting prowess, were difficult to live up to in real life, even for well-built males. Just as alcohol is used in 'straight society', barbiturates provided Skinheads with 'dutch courage', with the aggressive and violent style needed by any male who belonged to the skinhead subculture. They released inhibitions and aggression and reduced fear. Skinheads were willing to take on anybody when high on barbiturates, for pain hurt little, vision blurred and unable to see their opponents properly, they were not afraid of them.

It was not uncommon for Punks, when they tired of being Punks, to become Skinheads. Despite being the symbolic antithesis of Punk, they were both working-class in ethic and the Skinhead subculture and its espousal of 'conventional' traditional working-class society provided Punks with a symbolic medium for rejoining the conventional society they had totally rejected, as did their joint usage of barbiturates.

Punks would have been far less at home if they had become Mods or Rockabillies. Skinhead use of barbiturates was also attractive to barbiturate-using Punks. It was through the espousal of fighting that the erstwhile Punk integrated symbolically with conventional society. Being already users of barbiturates made taking part in fights so much easier.

The club-going scene

Tuinal was the substance most favoured by youngsters who participated in the club scene. Youngsters, according to Tyler (1988) in the Manchester club scene, would take amphetamine sulphate to fuel their furious jazz dancing: 'On the way home still charged up, they'll swallow a barb such as Tuinal, which allows them to present themselves back home in a credibly worn condition; they might even get some sleep in what remains of the night' (Tyler 1988: 105–6). They also took Tuinal for kicks. The excitement derived from dicing with death offered a powerful nihilist symbol for articulating their protest against their humdrum lives. A young local poet reported in the *New Musical Express* that 'children of 14, 15, 16 [were] hurtling headlong to death by their pathetic ignorant use of barbiturates, especially Tuinal .... They seem to regard this as some kind of test of street credibility, of how cool they can be. A hospital overdose bracelet is the latest fashion. They flirt with death as if it was nothing' (Tyler 1988: 108).

Barb Freaks

Piccadilly, and the West End in general, was a major centre where heavy barbiturate users congregated. They appeared in 1979–82 to be typical of London 'Barb Freaks' as they came from all over London, particularly South London, as well as the provinces. Most people who used barbiturates there, if not already heavy users when they joined the scene, soon became so. Apart from alcohol, barbiturates were often the primary or only substance used. The barbiturate user ranged in age from teenage to middle aged. The latter included long-term chronic DDU or ex-DDU patients. They supported their habits from social security benefits, if scripted, by selling part of their methadone scripts. Also by obtaining prescriptions from medical sources, occasionally by mugging or 'running' and prostitution. The latter included rent boys and a trans-sexual 'girl'. The heavy using 'Barb Freaks' mostly lived in squats or were homeless living on the streets. Some spent an occasional night in a hostel, e.g. Bruce House.

Once they started to use barbiturates regularly, the rapidity with which physical dependence and its social consequences takes hold and takes its toll played a major role in their becoming predominantly barbiturate users and spiralling into chaotic, homeless problem users.

The preference in Piccadilly for barbiturates was due not only to their physical effects, but the social and symbolic use to which they could be put. They fitted in with what Stimson (1973) has referred to as the 'junkie' type of addict. For most of them participation in the drug scene and social side of drug taking was just as important as the physical effects of the drugs they used. Involvement in the 'Dilly' drug scene gave them identity, meaning and purpose in life and a network of friends. Their life focused around the 'Dilly' and they spent much of their time there when not in hospital or prison.

Many barbiturate addicts who went into City Roads between 1978 and 1981 frequented Piccadilly and a survey of 80 of them (Jamieson et al., 1984: 82–91) indicates that, like the Punks and Skinheads, the majority came from disadvantaged and disrupted family backgrounds, e.g. neglected council estates, large families, paternal absenteeism, alcoholism or mental disturbance. They also fitted in with Stimson's 'junkie' stereotype.

The tranquillising and dulling effects of barbiturates offered Piccadilly barbiturate users an escape from the psychologically destructive effects of their social backgrounds and homeless chaotic lives on the street. Like the Punks they often referred to barbiturates' effects as enabling them to get 'fucking out of it'. They enabled them to sleep away their negative dispossessed lifestyles as well as allowing them to get a good night's sleep on the street or, if they strategically overdosed in the right place (and most knew their tolerance levels), a good night's sleep in the local hospital Casualty Department. Men and women who became prostitutes, including those who were opiate addicts, if not already taking Tuinal, often moved on to them to dull the psychological pain of their work, and not infrequently spiralled into chaotic problem use where they could only afford barbiturates.

In the status-conscious addict community, the chaotic dishevelled cheap drug-using 'Barb Freak' provided a symbolic status demarcator and was attributed the lowest status. Their appearance and lifestyle highlighted and reinforced the high status attached to the stable addict with a conventional appearance and lifestyle who could afford an expensive opiate habit. Within such a status-conscious community, living the lifestyle of the lowly 'Barb Freak' was also attractive to some with already low self-esteem as it justified and reinforced their sense of inadequacy and worthlessness.

Policy implications

The barbiturate 'epidemic' had major social and health implications. As Jamieson et al. (1984) pointed out, it provided a great deal of insight into British drug policy and its response to changing drug patterns and the significant contribution that practitioners and research have made in government policy making. It had a major influence on the development and structuring of drug services and practitioners' views on their goals and methods.

The barbiturate problem rapidly came to the attention of policy makers. From the early 1970s, medical practitioners in the drug field, and Casualty medical and nursing staff such as David Williams (1981) and Beryl Rose (1975) (who kept an eight-year register of drug overdoses) at the Middlesex Hospital, and street agencies articulated their concern publicly. They were particularly vocal in their agitation for a solution to the barbiturate problem and the need to control barbiturates.

The attaching of DDUs to London University Medical Schools served as a catalyst to the expansion of drug dependency research in the 1970s and the extensive research carried out during the barbiturate 'epidemic', particularly the survey by Ghodse (1976, 1977) of 62 London Casualty Departments certainly focused professional attention. Additionally, as the mortality and

Table 6.1 Barbiturate-related deaths among notified addicts 1967–93 (*n* = 316 deaths)

Year	Number of deaths	(% of all notified addict deaths)
1967	2	(17%)
1968	6	(50%)
1969	9	(32%)
1970	17	(53%)
1971	15	(58%)
1972	36	(69%)
1973	21	(60%)
1974	19	(50%)
1975	27	(49%)
1976	23	(43%)
1977	21	(41%)
1978	25	(37%)
1979	17	(30%)
1980	16	(25%)
1981	9	(12%)
1982	6	(6%)
1983	8	(7%)
1984	8	(11%)
1985	7	(9%)
1986	7	(6%)
1987	7	(5%)
1988	3	(2%)
1989	1	(1%)
1990	2	(1%)
1991	1	(<1%)
1992	2	(1%)
1993	1	(<1%)

Adapted from data originally presented in: Ghodse, H., Oyefeso, A. and Kilpatrick, B. (1998). 'Mortality of drug addicts in the United Kingdom 1967–1993', *International Journal of Epidemiology*, 27, 473–8.

morbidity statistics became available, these revealed, only too clearly, the nature and extent of the problem. CURB, the Campaign on the Use and Restriction of Barbiturates, which ran from 1975–77, was set up by a group of concerned doctors. It aimed to get doctors to voluntarily restrict their barbiturate prescribing. However, it was launched at a time when doctors were already switching to 'safer' tranquillisers, and barbiturate prescriptions were already declining in number. As a result, Banks and Waller (1988: 65) have questioned the campaign's effectiveness. At the same time the Committee on the Review of Medicines also examined barbiturates and in 1979 advocated severe restrictions on their usage. However, as can be inferred from Tyler (1988: 104–5), it was not legal controls that killed off barbiturate misuse, but the marketing of 'superior' tranquillisers (e.g. Valium and Librium) which pharmaceutical companies preferred to manufacture as they were more expensive and offered them greater profits.

Jamieson *et al.* (1984: 13) have pointed out that the debate in general in the social provision field in the 1970s began to centre on those in special need. In the drug field, the problem barbiturate user and the young homeless multiple substance misuser, became centres of attention. They were seen as exhibiting a new pattern of behaviour and a new problem needing new types of service. By the mid-1970s, multiple drug misuse came to be recognised by the government as a major drug addiction problem in Britain.

Multiple drug users, particularly problem users and the barbiturate problem in general, laid the groundwork for future services and the continuing debate today, within both the medical and voluntary sectors as to how services should be organised, particularly with regard to the problem user and their respective roles in it. It provided, too, an arena for articulating drug field rivalries, especially between the statutory agencies and non-statutory agencies.

One of the reasons the DDUs were set up in 1968 was to control the size of the drug addict population through prescribing policies (for fuller consideration, see Chapter 2, Volume II, by Philip Connell and John Strang). But the DDUs could not perform this function with regard to the barbiturate addict and multiple substance misuser as their brief was generally seen as applicable only to the opiates. The 'Barb Freak' epidemic brought home to them the difficulties of handling disruptive, often aggressive, non-compliant addicts within a medical setting. It led them to rethink their policies and introduce measures for handling them. The physical complications resulting from injecting barbiturates gave further impetus to the DDUs' move in the 1970s to supplying oral methadone rather than injectables.

The birth of City Roads

Street agencies were seeing many multiple drug users – particularly the young chaotic homeless user who had no contact with the DDUs. In a survey carried out by the Standing Conference on Drug Abuse (SCODA) (Jamieson *et al.* 1984: 16) in 1973, about half those seen by street agencies, about 200, had no contact with specialist medical agencies such as DDUs. This became a focus of rivalry between the street agencies and the DDUs. It was felt that the DDUs were too medically focused, prescribing only opioids and with long waiting lists, and that they did not offer emergency crisis intervention facilities. As a consequence they were not able to deal with the needs of this new young disruptive client group and it was argued that a specialist crisis centre outside the DDU services was needed to deal with them.

SCODA, the umbrella organisation for voluntary organisations, was set up in 1971. The barbiturate problem provided the voluntary sector with a rationale and a vehicle for making itself heard, with a basis for consolidating its position and expanding its power base. One of its first acts was to bring the barbiturate problem to the attention of the DHSS and agitate for specialised services for young problem users, particularly barbiturate misusers. The proceedings of a conference held by SCODA in 1977, reveal the views of the voluntary sector and the nature of the rivalry between the statutory and non-statutory sectors.

As a response to the extensive agitation, City Roads, the short-stay residential crisis intervention centre for chaotic problem users, funded partly by the DHSS, was eventually set up in 1978. Its history and social organisation have been described by Jamieson *et al.* (1984). According to their study, it was run mainly by social workers and nurses, with a psychiatric input, under the directorship of a social worker. Its multi-disciplinary approach and crisis-treatment focus was innovative and provided a testing ground for the multi-disciplinary approach, the role that social workers should play in rehabilitation and their position *vis-à-vis* the medical profession. It was monitored over a three-year period by Jamieson *et al.* (1984). This study was the first of its kind in the UK, providing the ground work and standards for the monitoring of drug projects later.

Being run by a social worker, City Roads enhanced the status of social workers and gave the voluntary organisations, mostly staffed by social workers, more political clout. City Roads became a significant player in the drugs field and spearheaded and helped pave the way for the expansion of the voluntary sector that took place in the 1980s (see Chapter 15).

Despite the government being aware from an early date of the extent of the barbiturate misuse problem, as David Turner (1994: 226) has pointed out (see Chapter 15, this volume), City Roads was set up after the problem was already beginning to disappear. In fact, within a couple of years, the number of their clients misusing barbiturates declined radically. Heroin had become cheap and easily available by the beginning of the 1980s which led to a new wave of problem heroin users and City Roads took over the role of providing crisis management for them instead. Finally, in 1985, barbiturates became a controlled drug under the Misuse of Drugs Act, in category B, the same category as cannabis, by which time the barbiturate problem was over.

Conclusions

Grant (1994) sees the British System as 'the story of a pragmatic and shifting response to a rapidly changing phenomenon'. Pragmatism is a highly valued virtue in British society, but the British System's pragmatic response to the barbiturate 'epidemic' is more accurately and meaningfully seen as an example of the shortcomings of such a system. It reflects the inability of a system without a coherent clear-cut policy to respond quickly to the changing patterns of drug use.

City Roads demonstrates the drawbacks of a government policy where there is no pre-existing mechanism for responding rapidly to new patterns and problems of drug misuse and where getting things changed and new services introduced is often left to motivated individuals pressuring local and central government. As Jamieson *et al.* (1984) make clear, it was a six-year uphill task getting City Roads established. It was due to a number of committed individuals bringing pressure to bear on the government and local funding organisations and a number of people at the DHSS who were favourably disposed to the proposed project and who worked inside the Government Health Department to secure the necessary support and funding.

A major lesson learnt from City Roads and the barbiturate problem, is the need for central and local government to have coherent policies which can quickly respond to changing drug patterns and problems and can immediately fund and introduce the new services needed.

It also reinforces once again the truism in the drug field that when one drug is controlled, another will take its place. The government did not immediately learn from the barbiturate problem, for tranquillisers took the place of barbiturates. They became extensively misused too, and once again it was several years before the government took any action. The lesson that needs to be learnt from the barbiturate problem is that the misuse potential of all new psychotropic drugs should be extensively monitored and responded to as soon as they come on to the market.

References

Banks, A. and Waller, T. A. N., 1988, *Drug Misuse: A Practical Handbook for GPs*, Blackwell, Oxford.

Bewley, T. H., 1966, Recent Changes in the Pattern of Drug Abuse in the United Kingdom, *Bulletin on Narcotics*, 18, 4, 1–13.

Burr, A., 1983, The Piccadilly Drug Scene, *British Journal of Addiction*, 78, 1, 5–19.

Burr, A., 1984a, The Illicit Non-Pharmaceutical Heroin Market and Drug Scene in Kensington Market, *British Journal of Addiction*, 79, 3, 337–43.

Burr, A., 1984b, The Ideologies of Despair: A Symbolic Interpretation of Punks and Skinheads Usage of Barbiturates, *Social Science and Medicine*, 19, 9, 929–38.

Committee on the Review of Medicines, 1979, Recommendations on Barbiturate Preparations, *British Medical Journal*, 2, 719–20.

D'Orban, P. T., 1976, Barbiturate Abuse, *Journal of Medical Ethics*, 2, 63–7.

Forrest, J. A. H. and Tarala, R. A., 1973, Abuse of Drugs for 'Kicks': A Review of 252 Admissions, *British Medical Journal*, 4, 136–9.

Ghodse, A. H., 1976, Drug Problems Dealt with by 62 London Casualty Departments, *British Journal of Preventive and Social Medicine*, 30, 251–6.

Ghodse, A. H., 1977, Drug Dependent Individuals Dealt with by London Casualty Departments, *British Journal of Psychiatry*, 131, 273–80.

Ghodse, A. H., 1979, Recommendations by Accident and Emergency Staff about Drug-Overdose Patients, *Social Science and Medicine*, 13A, 169–73.

Ghodse, A. H. and Rawson, N. S., 1978a, Distribution of Drug-Related Problems among London Casualty Departments, *British Journal of Psychiatry*, 132, 467–72.

Ghodse, A. H., Sheehan, M., Stevens, B., Taylor, C. and Edwards, G., 1978b, Mortality amongst Addicts in Greater London, *British Medical Journal*, 2, 1742–4.

Ghodse, A. H., Oyefeso, A. and Kilpatrick, B., 1998, Mortality of Drug Addicts in the United Kingdom, 1962–1993, *International Journal of Epidemiology*, 27, 3, 473–8.

Grant, M., 1994, Foreword: What is so Special about the British System?, in Strang, J. and Gossop, M. (eds) *Heroin Addiction and Drug Policy: The British System*, Oxford University Press, Oxford.

Hall, S. and Jefferson, T. (eds), 1976, *Resistance Through Rituals: Youth Subcultures in Post-War Britain*, Hutchinson, London, Centre for Contemporary Cultural Studies, University of Birmingham.

Hebdige, D., 1979, *Subculture: The Meaning of Style*, Methuen, London.

Institute for the Study of Drug Dependence, 1979, Barbiturates – From Valuable Medicine to Dangerous Drug, *Drug Link*, Spring, 11, 5–7.

Jamieson, A., Glanz, A. and MacGregor, S., 1984, *Dealing with Drug Misuse: Crisis Intervention in the City*, Tavistock, London.

Mitchell, B. and Rose, B., 1975, Barbiturate Abuse – A Growing Problem, *Nursing Times*, 18 September, 1488–90.

Mitcheson, M., 1994, Drug Clinics in the 1970s, in Strang, J. and Gossop, M. (eds) *Heroin Addiction and Drug Policy: The British System*, Oxford University Press, Oxford, 178–91.

Mitcheson, M., Davidson, J. and Hawks, D., 1971, Sedative Abuse by Heroin Addicts, *Journal of Psychedelic Drugs*, 4, 2, 123–31.

Mitcheson, M., Davidson, J., Hawkes, D., Hitchens, C. and Malone, S., 1970, Sedative Abuse by Heroin Addicts, *Lancet*, 1, 606–7.

Stevens, B., 1978, Deaths of Drug Addicts in London during 1970–74: Toxicological, Legal and Demographic Findings, *Medicine, Science and the Law*, April, 18, 2, 128–37.

Stimson, G. V., 1973, *Heroin and Behaviour, Diversity among Addicts Attending London Clinics*, Irish University Press, Shannon.

Strang, J. and Gossop, M. (eds), 1994, *Heroin Addiction and Drug Policy: The British System*, Oxford University Press, Oxford.

Teff, H., 1975, *Drugs, Society and the Law*, Saxon House, Farnborough.

Teggin, A. F. and Bewley, T. H., 1979, Withdrawal Treatment for Barbiturate Dependence, *The Practitioner*, 223, 1333, 106–7.

Turner, B., 1984, *The Body and Society, Explorations in Social Theory*, Basil Blackwell, Oxford.

Turner, D., 1994, The Development of the Voluntary Sector: No Further Need for Pioneers?, in J. Strang and M. Gossop (eds) *Heroin Addiction and Drug Policy: The British System*, Oxford University Press, Oxford, 222–30.

Tyler, A., 1988, *Street Drugs: The Facts Explained, the Myths Exploded*, New English Library, Hodder & Stoughton, London.

Williams, D., 1981, The Problem in a Central London Hospital, in R. Murray, A. H. Ghodse, C. Harris, D. Williams and P. Williams (eds) *The Misuse of Psychotropic Drugs*, Gaskell, London, 55–88.

Chapter 7

Heroin epidemics and social exclusion in the UK, 1980–2000

Howard Parker

Introduction

During the early 1980s widespread heroin use was found, for the first time, in many UK cities and nearby towns. Estimates of the numbers involved during the mid-1980s vary between 100 and 150 thousand users (in Scotland, England and Wales, as Northern Ireland was unaffected). The social profile of these new users was remarkably consistent. They were from the social margins. One of the most detailed studies during this period was undertaken in Wirral, Merseyside, in N.W. England. This chapter re-describes and updates the key findings of this four-year study (see Parker *et al.*, 1988) but situates them in the broader epidemiology of heroin outbreaks or 'epidemics'.

With increasing evidence that a second wave of heroin outbreaks may be developing in the UK what we learnt during the 1980s takes on renewed significance. On the other hand the outline 'model' of re-emergence of heroin uptake in youth populations in England and Scotland at the end of the 1990s is already deviating from the 1980s profile of susceptibility. The immediate challenge is to assess the value of our accepted wisdom, built on the first epidemic and its longer-term consequences, against what is currently unfolding.

The Wirral outbreak

Scope of the research

Wirral on Merseyside (population 340,000 in 1980) became one of the numerous unexpected sites of a full-scale heroin outbreak which began around 1979 and the impact of which has lasted for well over a decade. A government-funded four-year study (e.g. Parker *et al.*, 1988; Chadwick and Parker, 1988) attempted to produce a comprehensive picture of the impact of this outbreak on users, their families, the wider community and unusually on the 'bewildered' range of local officials charged with developing official responses to an unprecedented drugs problem.

A clutch of interweaving research techniques was used ranging from observation in professional meetings to interviewing users and dealers and undertaking a longitudinal three-part capture–recapture or multi-enumeration analysis of all heroin users known to ten key agencies. This was supplemented by a 'snowball' study into the 'hidden' sector of users not known to local agencies. A study of the linkage between the unprecedented rise in recorded acquisitive crime rates (e.g. burglary) and this heroin outbreak was also undertaken (e.g. Parker and Newcombe, 1987).

The patterns and profiles

The 'capturing' of heroin users as they moved in and out of the criminal justice system (police records, probation service) treatment or counselling (Home Office Notifications Index, DDUs, Drugs Council, GPs, Psychiatric Units) and local authority services (Social Services Department, Education Department) over three years identified around 1,300 'known' users in the mid-1980s, with over 2,000 unique individuals having been identified by 1988. However, after the hidden sector study it was concluded at least 4,000 young adult users were residing in the Wirral.

The dominant profile (Parker et al., 1987) of these new users was male (initial ratio 3.6:1, but eventually 2:1). The modal age was 19, the peak age range 18–22 years with 16–30 years covering over 92 per cent of the whole user population. Over 86 per cent of users available for employment were in fact unemployed as against a then very high 20 per cent regional rate. Over half had no educational qualifications and few even had 'O' levels upon finishing secondary school education. The vast majority were daily heroin users who 'chased the dragon' before gradually moving to injecting, particularly through the late 1980s. Users typically had daily habits of 0.25–0.5 gm per day but a minority were using in excess of a gram a day.

A key finding was that this population came from families that lived in the borough's most socially deprived area. A 'social malaise' analysis of the townships in which they predominantly lived found very high correlations between the residential address and unemployment, council housing tenancies, overcrowding, three or more children in the household, unskilled employment, single parenting and no access to a car (Parker et al., 1987).

It also became clear that whilst there were some 'middle-class' communities and individuals affected by the diffusion of this outbreak, there was a strong linkage between youth, 'problematic' heroin use and a cluster of socio-economic malaise indicators, today referred to as *social exclusion*. This connection which is found repeatedly in British 'problem' drug users (ACMD, 1998) remained robust right across the four years of investigation.

The effect on the community

The grassroots development of several parents', predominantly mothers', self-help groups (Dorn *et al.*, 1987; Parker and Donnelly, 1990) bore witness to the tensions that families 'hosting' a young heroin user were under. With teenage sons stealing from home, 'going missing' and being responsible for unwanted visits from unpaid heroin dealers large numbers of families had to either learn to live with a heroin user or through time put more distance between user and family home. As their drugs careers unfolded some young men and women left home and attempted to live elsewhere including, for many, periods in Remand Centres and local prisons.

A steady flow (around 20 a year) of pregnant female heroin users also began to emerge. This triggered considerable tension in hospital maternity units, where these young women were subjected to overt criticism and resultant stigma. Over a hundred 'cases' were identified during the mid-1980s (see also Klenka, 1986). Child protection agencies also had to make difficult assessments about parenting. Interestingly the vast majority of heroin babies were not taken into care. Instead, community-based care 'contracts' were made primarily with maternal grandmothers who supported their heroin-using daughters with child care and informal supervision (Parker *et al.*, 1988).

Acquisitive crime rose dramatically during this period. Domestic burglaries for Wirral rose from 2,824 in 1979 to a recorded rate of 10,238 in 1986 and significant rises were found for theft from vehicles and burglary of other premises. A detailed study comparing the identity codes of known heroin users with police and court records and interviewing users showed that most of these increases were a direct consequence of young adult heroin users committing specifically acquisitive crime to fund their heroin habits. Wirral's crime rate per head of population rose far more rapidly than elsewhere on Merseyside, including Liverpool, as a consequence of its heroin outbreak.

Further confirmation of the heroin–social exclusion linkage was found when the criminal careers of these daily heroin users were analysed. Whilst some had no criminal record prior to heroin use, the majority did have delinquent antecedents prior to onset. Heroin use produced an extension and amplification of a deviant life style rather than created it.

The epidemic model

One of the extraordinary features of the Wirral outbreak was that its initial 'epidemic' phase largely mimicked the elaborate model developed by the Americans based on their postwar inner city epidemics. The heroin epidemiologists (Hughes, 1977; Hunt and Chambers, 1976) treat heroin uptake rather like an infectious disease whereby a small group of susceptibles are present in the wider population. Those who will ever try heroin although a small minority nearly all initiate in a fixed period. This *incidence* (initiates or new cases) rises rapidly for about four years before peaking at a far higher rate than previously recorded. Incidence then starts to fall. For heroin use *prevalence* (number of users in the community by each year) is maintained at an even higher level for several years if, as is usually the case, most users do not give up (or indeed migrate or die) for several years.

This is almost exactly what happened on the Wirral although a brief review at the end of the 1980s (Newcombe and Parker, 1991) suggested that endemic prevalence levels remained higher than the original American model predicted, perhaps due to a switch to injecting and extensive methadone maintenance 'slowing down' abstinence or 'outcidence'. With other studies in the Scottish cities (Haw, 1985) and on the west side of Britain (Fazey, 1987; Gay *et al.*, 1985; Pearson *et al.*, 1986) suggesting similar outbreak cycles were under way right across the 1979–87 period we can see this time frame as defining the UK's first heroin epidemic. This said, we must also expect to find micro outbreaks unfolding outside this period (Ditton and Frischer, 1998).

One other salient feature of this working model was the distinction made between micro and macro diffusion. *Micro diffusion* involves spread through personal/social contact as more experienced users facilitate novices and the knowledge about price, purity, how to smoke, chase or inject, which feelings to look for, how to cope in emergencies, etc. are all passed on between associates. In a full-blown outbreak this diffusion occurs simultaneously on numerous sites where 'susceptible' populations reside. *Macro diffusion* involves geographical spread. The original model noted these outbreaks began in densely populated, typically 'inner city' environments then spread outwards to other urban communities and then beyond being likely to affect smaller towns several years down the line (Pearson *et al.*, 1986) Again this is what occurred on the Wirral. The borough is divided administratively into over 50 'townships' yet only six of these (certain 'notorious' deprived areas and 'problem' estates) accounted for over half the 'known' users, although other outer townships were indeed affected through time (Chadwick and Parker, 1988).

Significantly incidence, new cases emerging, also remained higher in the deprived 'six' heroin hotspots as both older and younger (than the mean) users eventually surfaced – most notably young women many of whom initiated via established using partners, family and friends (micro diffusion again). This in turn helped delay any downturn in prevalence. Consistent with the longevity of this outbreak was both the switch to injecting (a key stage in long-term dependence) and the move towards regular poly-drug use whereby cannabis, heroin and methadone (usually prescribed but also from the street market) were joined by illicit temazepam in particular.

However, it started to become clear around the 1986–88 period that the American model was becoming a less effective predictor. The main reason for this was that it assumed that the whole epidemic 'cycle' lasted little more than ten years. The incidence and prevalence curves were thus conceived as bell or 'half moon' shaped, although prevalence was acknowledged to settle at a higher endemic level. However, a brief follow-up of the Wirral situation (Newcombe and Parker, 1991) confirmed what had been suspected at the final capture–recapture of known users in 1988 – that whilst incidence had fallen sharply from nearly 800 cases in 1984–85 to around 260 in 1986–87 and down to less than 100 by 1990 – prevalence was not following as quickly as predicted (Chadwick and Parker, 1988).

Figure 7.1 is speculative. It is based on the 'known' users data multiplied by two (on the assumption that by the late 1980s the 'hidden' user population, which was estimated scientifically in 1986–87 to be over twice the size of the known user population was shrinking as more long-term users finally emerged for advice, treatment or were netted by the criminal justice system). It also abandons the ten-year 'cycle' notion. The incidence curve, arithmetically, in fact predicts nearly 6,000 initiates but we must remember that some 'initiates' do not become regular users, whilst others ('chippers') manage to use heroin only occasionally and recreationally.

The 'failure' of the prevalence rate to fall steeply even by the early 1990s is further supported by the current situation. Wirral's main drug service, for instance, has seen around 2,400 unique individuals over the 1990s and even in 1998 had around 1,400 service users/patients.[1] It may well be that if UK researchers had monitored the 1980s outbreaks more carefully we would

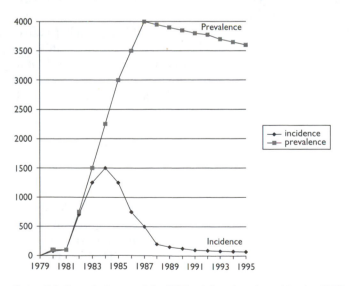

Figure 7.1 Speculative model of Wirral first heroin epidemic, 1979–95
Source: Author.

have found this prevalence rate 'shape' occurred in other outbreak areas, for instance as in Glasgow (Ditton and Frischer, 1998).

In conclusion, the Wirral heroin outbreak saw incidence rising steeply, peaking after four years then declining rapidly to a far lower endemic level. Prevalence has not fallen significantly, however, and remains stubbornly high as older users continue and a small but significant incidence rate is maintained even including second-generation initiates of the original early 1980s 'heroin families'. It cannot be proven but it seems likely that certain contingencies – such as the switch to injecting, the move to poly-drug use and the routine prescribing of diamorphine and methadone – will have encouraged this – whatever the considerable social gains methadone maintenance has brought to the Wirral community.

Heroin's 'return' at the end of the 1990s

Heroin use clearly remains endemic in many of the old sites such as Merseyside in N.W. England and Strathclyde in Scotland, given that many of those who started using in the 1980s continue with long-term combination drugs careers often including prescribed methadone. Moreover we have seen a continuing incidence 'trickle' from these old sites along with the last wave of 1980s outbreaks which also left precursors or heroin 'footprints' in cities like Bradford (Pearson and Patel, 1998) and towns in several English and Scottish regions which are now experiencing full-blown outbreaks. This said and compared with the 1980s, the first half of the 1990s has clearly been a quiet (endemic) period in respect of heroin.

However, signs of change have since emerged with increases in young users entering treatment around 1994–95 and with intelligence that far more heroin was being imported via the Balkan route across Europe into the UK, 'rumours' of new heroin spread patterns multiplied. They reached such a pitch by 1997 that the UK government commissioned a rapid audit of the situation in England and Wales (but alas not Scotland).

This 'early warning' enquiry painted a disturbing picture of the geographical spread of new heroin uptake (Parker et al., 1998a). A national postal survey of all Police Forces and Drug Action Teams (DATs) in England and Wales was undertaken with extensive follow-up telephone interviews all around the country and fieldwork visits in several areas hosting new outbreaks. By 'networking' with key informants, interviewing local professionals and young heroin users/dealers an outline national picture was built up, the cornerstone of which was over 200 separate survey returns. Eventually 73 per cent of DATs and 86 per cent of Police Forces made returns describing their local drugs scene. This provided outline information for about 90 per cent of the two countries.

The picture to emerge was unequivocal in respect of the geographical spread of new heroin outbreaks amongst young people (under 19s). Overall

80 per cent of DATs and 81 per cent of Police Forces making returns reported recent new clusters of young heroin users within their jurisdictions. Many were very small and only briefly described; however, in some cases significant established outbreaks were reported (e.g. Bristol, Bradford, Hull). Whilst non-returners are likely to represent 'no new outbreaks' this is still an unprecedented spread profile. The most significant finding in respect of comparisons with the 1980s epidemic was that the new spread was primarily in areas with no appreciable heroin history (e.g. Eastern England, West Midlands, much of Yorkshire). This said those areas – small cities – with current full-scale outbreaks which began around 1993–94 had heroin 'foot-prints' from the 1980s. In short their outbreaks are already full blown because heroin precursors (e.g. availability) were present in these cities from the end of the last epidemic.

Another key finding was that the old heroin regions, particularly Mersey-side, are not reporting significant new heroin uptake but instead are now the 'kilo' wholesale depots for heroin distribution to new markets with the motorway networks playing a key role in communication and transportation. This is a modification of macro diffusion in postmodern times whereby the spread from the old city sites to neighbouring areas is not the norm. Instead, with geographical distance no longer a constraint and motorways and mobile phones becoming the ideal communication aids, the new areas affected are often well away from any cities or 'old' heroin sites. This, as we will see, also links to youthful susceptibility.

Heroin, youth and social exclusion?

During the early 1990s a 'post-heroin' generation of recreational drug users emerged. The UK has the highest proportion of young 'recreational' drug users in Europe (EMCDDA, 1998). The use of the ubiquitous cannabis, LSD, amphetamines, ecstasy and 'poppers' has dominated the drugs rep-ertoires of 1990s youth (Parker et al., 1998). Those who were teenagers in the first half of the decade almost universally eschewed heroin, crack cocaine and the 'injecting' of any illicit substance. However, behind them has come another age cohort who being unable to remember the 1980s and that 'heroin screws you up' and that needle sharing spreads HIV/AIDS – have no real cognisance of the lessons from the first epidemic. They may have become 'drugwise' but based on experiences of largely non-addictive drugs which they use only occasionally (Parker et al., 1998). Thus when heroin is re-marketed as 'brown' as smokable and in £5 and £10 wraps and particularly to youth populations, without any collective awareness about the dangers and dependency-creating potential of heroin, we should not be surprised by a significant uptake. Moreover, if these new markets are being purposefully made in towns with no heroin history and far away from cities which have, then we have a considerable modification on the epidemiology of the first

UK epidemic. However, the fundamental question must be concerned with whether the new heroin outbreaks will once again be directly related to socio-economic malaise or what is now called social exclusion. Will the profile of these new young heroin triers and users be of young people living in relative poverty, in rundown neighbourhoods who have not done well at school, tend to be delinquent and have poor outcomes in terms of obtaining legitimate employment? In short, will social exclusion be the primary context definer of the second wave and thus also in a sense contain the outbreak as in the 1980s? The even worse scenario is that with such sophisticated supply-led remarketing and with such a drug experienced yet 'susceptible' youth population – that smoking brown will become acceptable at the serious end of the recreational drugs scene and thus move well beyond the social exclusion zones.

The answers to this key question are not yet fully available. The picture to emerge from the audit was that age of heroin onset is now far younger. Over a third of the survey returns identified 'under 16s' as one age band involved in their area. With the age of onset of all drug trying falling (McKeganey and Norrie, 1999; Aldridge et al., 1999) we must, this time, see 14–25 being the 'at risk' age band. The dominance of 'smoking' found in the early stages of the first epidemic is being repeated. However, in those areas which are 3–4 years into their outbreak the beginnings of a switch to injecting were reported. The over 3:1 male to female ratio was also the norm. Again this was found in the 1980s followed by later incidence amongst more women whereby the final ratio moved towards 2:1. On the other hand there is significant involvement amongst Asian youth reported this time around which was largely absent during the 1980s.

Turning to the socio-economic profile, the dominant descriptions offered by survey returns was still of socially excluded youth being at the core of the local 'problem'. So even in affected towns heroin use was predominantly sited in the area's poorest housing clusters or 'estates'. This said, a significant minority of reporters challenged this profile, insisting that the picture was far more complex and involved 'bonded' more conventional and affluent young people. With reports of heroin being used as a post-clubbing 'chill-out' drug and of 'respectable' parents contacting helplines and local drugs services disclosing their teenage children were taking heroin, the audit suggests a scenario of heroin use extending beyond the social exclusion definers found in the 1980s.

Finally with routine school-based surveys during the first half of the 1990s finding less than 1 per cent of respondents reporting heroin trying, the fact that in-school adolescents are now disclosing trying at 2–4 per cent in Northern England (Aldridge et al., 1999); and urban Scotland (McKeganey and Norrie, 1999) offers a picture of greater penetration into 'included' more conventional youth populations. Certainly there is sufficient 'intuitive' evidence here to make the further testing of this new spread and penetration hypothesis a priority.

Conclusion

The heroin outbreaks which were part of the UK's first epidemic during the 1980s, seriously affected N.W. England, London, many towns on the west of Britain and the Scottish cities. These outbreaks had a 'classic' epidemiology and certainly the epidemic phase largely mimicked those modelled in the USA during the 1960s and 1970s. Susceptible youth who took up heroin proved to be those living in socially deprived urban areas who had few educational qualifications, were unemployed and who tended to have 'delinquent careers' prior to the onset of heroin use at about 18–21 years of age. As their heroin use became dependent use most turned to acquisitive crime, drug dealing and, for some women, the sex industry to help fund increasingly expensive habits (0.25–0.5 gm heroin a day). Many young men became entangled in the criminal justice system and heroin 'mothers' became a key concern for statutory child care agencies. On the Wirral the number of users in the borough each year (prevalence) remained stubbornly high into the 1990s, well after the number of initiates (incidence) began to fall. The switch from smoking to injecting, which occurred during the parallel HIV/AIDS epidemic period, was however very well managed in that the public health strategies (methadone, needle exchanges, outreach services, media messages) were highly successful is preventing HIV spread. On the other hand, we will probably never know whether the extensive methadone maintenance programmes unintentionally prolonged the opiate careers of this heroin generation. Certainly a large proportion of them have remained on prescribed methadone for very many years.

This raises the key point about whether the primary treatment regime for the new users of any second epidemic should be methadone prescribing. There are undoubted benefits from methadone maintenance in terms of stabilising lifestyles, reducing crime and levels of illicit drug use in patients. However, whether such a youthful population should be subjected to this regime is another matter given how dependent so many of the first wave have become on their 'meth'. Moreover, with the strong tendency for combination or poly-drug use to become the norm at the heavy end of drug-use careers it may well be that prescribed methadone, even administered under supervision in 'swallow clinics', could well be misused. The danger is that if prescribed very early in a 'teenage' heroin career it becomes an addition to rather than an alternative to poly-drug use.

The UK enters the new millennium with a complex and serious drugs problem – the re-emergence of heroin in sections of its youth population. Whilst the recreational drugs scene amongst 1990s youth was regarded by adult worlds as *the* drugs problem, this normalised self-regulated drug trying and use has not been based on particularly physically 'addictive' drugs and the casualty rate has been relatively small. Heroin is far less forgiving. Fifteen years ago and for tens of thousands of young Britons from the social margins, heroin began as a solution and ended up a problem. If we are seeing a second heroin epidemic then this time around we at least already have an 'early warning'. Moreover, based on what we learnt from heroin outbreaks of the 1980s we may also have an outline notion of what is likely to unfold in the new heroin hotspots. Yet over a decade on, the whole drugs backcloth is very different and today's youth have a distinctive, collective drugs wisdom and so we also have a sense that these new young 'brown' users will, in turn, in time, write a new chapter in heroin epidemiology.

Acknowledgements

Thanks to Geoff Pearson and Jason Ditton for some good ideas and to the now Merseyside Drugs Prevention Initiative for permission to quote from an unpublished report.

Note

1 With special thanks to Dr Stefan Janickiewicz, Director of Wirral Drugs Service.

References

ACMD (1998). *Drug Misuse and the Environment*. Advisory Council on the Misuse of Drugs, Home Office, London.

Aldridge, J., Parker, H. and Measham, F. (1999). *Drug Trying and Drug Use Across Adolescence*. Home Office Drugs Prevention Initiative, Home Office, London.

Chadwick, C. and Parker, H. (1988). *Wirral's Enduring Heroin Problem: The Prevalence, Incidence and Characteristics of Drug Use in Wirral 1984–7*. Misuse of Drugs Research Project, Liverpool University.

Ditton, J. and Frischer, M. (1998). *Computerised Projection of Future Heroin Epidemics: A Necessity for the 21st Century?* University of Sheffield (unpublished).

Dorn, N. *et al.* (1987). *Coping with a Nightmare: Family Feelings about Long Term Drug Use*. ISDD, London.

EMCDDA (1998). *Annual Report: Drug Problems in the European Union*. European Monitoring Centre for Drugs and Drug Addiction, Lisbon.

Fazey, C. (1987). *The Evaluation of the Liverpool Drug Dependency Clinic 1985–87*. Mersey Regional Health, Liverpool.

Gay, M. *et al.* (1985). *The Interim Report*. Avon Drug Abuse Monitoring Project, Hartcliffe Health Centre, Bristol.

Haw, S. (1985). *Drug Problems in Greater Manchester*. SCODA, Glasgow.

Hughes, P. (1977). *Behind the Wall of Respect*. University of Chicago Press, Chicago.

Hunt, L. and Chambers, C. (1976). *The Heroin Epidemics: A Study of Heroin Use in the United States*. Spectrum, New York.

Klenka, H. (1986). 'Babies Born in a District General Hospital to Mothers Taking Heroin'. *British Medical Journal*, 293: 745–6.

McKeganey, N. and Norrie, J. (1999). 'Pre-teen Drug Misuse in Scotland'. *Addiction Research*, 7: 493–507.

Newcombe, R. and Parker, H. (1991). *Drug Misuse in Wirral: An Endemic Problem?* Report to the (Wirral) Home Office Drugs Prevention Team (unpublished).

Parker, H. and Newcombe, R. (1987). 'Heroin Use and Acquisitive Crime in an English Community'. *British Journal of Sociology*, 38: 331–50.

Parker, H. and Donnelly, L. (1990). 'Parents, Self Help and Heroin Use'. *Druglink*, July, 5, 4: 8–10.

Parker, H., Newcombe, R. and Bakx, K. (1987). 'The New Heroin Users: Prevalence and Characteristics in Wirral, Merseyside'. *British Journal of Addiction*, 82, 147–57.

Parker, H., Bakx, K. and Newcombe, R. (1988). *Living with Heroin: The Impact of a Heroin Epidemic on an English Community*. Open University Press, Buckingham.

Parker, H., Aldridge, J. and Measham, F. (1998). *Illegal Leisure: The Normalisation of Adolescent Recreational Drug Use*. Routledge, London.

Parker, H., Egginton, R. and Bury, C. (1998a). *New Heroin Outbreaks amongst Young People in England and Wales*. Police Research Group, Crime Detection and Prevention Series, Paper 92, Home Office, London.

Pearson, G. and Patel, K. (1998). 'Drugs, Deprivation and Ethnicity: Outreach amongst Asian Drug Users in a Northern English city'. *Journal of Drug Issues*, 28: 199–224.

Pearson, G., Gilman, M. and McIver, S. (1986). *Young People and Heroin: An Examination of Heroin Use in the North of England*. Health Education Council, London.

Chapter 8

Flexible hierarchies and dynamic disorder

The trading and distribution of illicit heroin in Britain and Europe

Roger Lewis

(This chapter originally appeared in J. Strang and M. Gossop (eds) *Heroin Addiction and Drug Policy; The British System*, Oxford University Press 1994.)

Introduction

Some profound changes have occurred in heroin consumption in Britain and Europe over the past quarter of a century. Most traces of the 'alternative' ideology of the early 1970s have disappeared. The icon/role model of the misunderstood 'right-on' street junkie/anti-hero, surviving on his own terms against an oppressive society, has lost its attraction. By the mid-1980s heroin use had become an almost banal affair, with dwindling transgressive status. Growing awareness of the risks of human immuno-deficiency virus (HIV) infection has also affected attitudes. Yet, despite high rates of social marginalization, familial rejection, violence, arrest, prison, overdose, relapse and seropositivity, a proportion of the addict population hang on tenaciously to their lives, their drugs and their battered identities. Others lead relatively ordinary lives of work or study in which their drug use is secret, or known only to their families and close friends. The everyday nature of such consumption contributes to its 'invisibility'.

Generally speaking, the illicit market in heroin has remained resilient, although polydrug use tends to be the norm for most consumers. Where heroin has become hard to obtain, it has been replaced by pharmaceutical preparations, such as dihydrocodeine, buprenorphine and benzodiazepine in cities such as Nottingham and Edinburgh. Changes in the supply and marketing of heroin and other illicit drugs cannot be understood without taking account of productive origin, trading routes, local and regional geography, and drug-related entrepreneurial crime. Similarly, demand for drugs cannot be understood if the social formation, economic situation and cultural predispositions of the consumer population are ignored. The availability of drugs and a social network within which drug users socialize are as critical to the development of a market as the simple presence of individuals predisposed to drug use. Evidence from the United Kingdom suggests that when social and supply networks are absent such individuals are unlikely to become involved in illicit drug use, at least within their own community (de Alarcon 1973; Mott and Rathod 1976; Fraser and George 1988).

The study of illicit drug markets is still in its infancy. Most of the early work originated in the United States (Preble and Casey 1969; Redlinger 1974; Johnson *et al.* 1985). Since then, a pool of epidemiological and ethnographic knowledge has evolved in several European countries. A number of studies have attempted to examine how distribution takes place, the manner in which transactions are negotiated, and the way illicit heroin markets function (Ingold 1984; Lewis *et al.* 1985; Dorn and South 1987; Fraser and George 1988; Power 1990; Arlacchi and Lewis 1990a,b).

A growing market and its components

There has been an illicit market in heroin in Britain since the mid-1960s when six pharmaceutical heroin pills (each containing 10 mg) could be purchased for £1. Although so-called 'Chinese' heroin was evident in London prior to 1968 when the treatment system was restructured, a firmly rooted market in illicitly imported heroin did not develop until the early 1970s. South-east Asian 'No. 3' smoking heroin (30–45 per cent purity) and 'No. 4' or 'Thai' heroin (50–70 per cent purity) were largely supplanted in the late 1970s when illicit heroin manufactured in South-west Asia came on stream. This ranged from crudely refined, chocolate-coloured heroin from Iran, first seen in London in 1974, to beige or buff-coloured Turkish, Pakistani and Afghan heroin. The years 1978–80 were a watershed for heroin use in Britain, and Western Europe generally. Increased availability and falling prices filled existing demand, encouraged experimentation, and generated new demand. There was a decline in subcultural taboos against heroin and a concurrent spread in consumption to provincial towns and cities (Lewis *et al.* 1985).

Retail heroin was dealt initially in the centres of major cities. In due course dealing extended beyond the centres and beyond the cities themselves. This 'shift to the periphery' in which activity radiated outwards to the suburbs (particularly those districts displaying high indices of social deprivation), was evident in Paris by 1978 (C. Olivenstein, personal communication 1978) and in Rome by 1980 (Arlacchi and Lewis 1987). Whereas some pockets of squatted and short-life housing in London were displaying high rates of consumption by the mid-1970s, the extent of heroin use on inner-city and suburban estates was not generally acknowledged until 1982. Subsequent studies in the north of England and Scotland revealed widespread heroin use in local communities in Liverpool, Manchester, the Wirral, Glasgow and Edinburgh. These studies revealed that heroin consumption was not uniformly dispersed through given cities or regions, but tended to be concentrated in particular districts (Haw 1985; Parker *et al.* 1986; Pearson *et al.* 1987; Haw and Liddell 1989). Small sub-markets developed in these districts which in turn attracted novitiates, who had never participated in a central drug scene.

In the initial stages of the European market in the early 1970s, couriers would bring in multiple kilos of heroin by air from the Far East. The global nature and magnitude of the traffic by the 1980s was such that large numbers of trucks and freighters began to be intercepted carrying cargoes of heroin from the Near East, the Indian subcontinent and South-east Asia. Afghan, Pakistani, Turkish, Iranian and Middle Eastern heroin has tended to predominate in Western Europe over the last 10 years. Production capacity in South-west Asia remains high. Seven hundred and forty-one kilos of heroin were seized in Turkey alone in the first 6 months of 1989 (International Narcotics Control Board (INCB) 1989). In late 1990 over one-fifth of a ton was found in a single overland shipment entering Britain through the Channel ports.

With the establishment of a fully fledged market in Britain the number of heroin seizures by the police rose rapidly in the early 1980s, peaking at 3003 in 1985. They subsequently declined to 1877 seizures in 1987 and rose again in 1988. The quantity of heroin seized by HM Customs between 1980 and 1988 indicates a similar trend. Less than 50 kilos of heroin were seized by Customs in 1980, 334 kilos in 1985, 179 kilos in 1986, and 211 kilos in 1988 (Institute for the Study of Drug Dependence (ISDD) 1990). A European decline in overdose deaths, along with a fall in seizures, raised hopes that consumption might have peaked in 1986. However, a marked rise in heroin-related mortalities in the late 1980s (INCB 1989), probably related to increased heroin purity at street level and the spread of HIV, suggests that demand remains strong and supplies are available.

The retail purity of illicit heroin in Britain and Holland has always been relatively high compared with the United States, where an organized crime presence fostered dilution practices and lowered customer expectations. The size and poverty of the United States' addict population may have resulted in larger numbers attempting 'to live off the market' by heavily diluting the product before trading it forward. In Britain long-established commercial, colonial, and cultural ties with a number of heroin-producing nations enabled illicit entrepreneurs to take advantage of favourable trading terms. Some of the benefits (lower price and higher purity) were passed on to the consumer. In the early 1980s, the purity of retail heroin in London was sometimes as high as 45–55 per cent (Lewis *et al.* 1985). Average retail purity in Britain was 39 per cent in 1985, 30 per cent in 1987, and 38 per cent in 1989 (ISDD 1990). Such purities have been consistently higher than in some other European countries, which are experiencing rising overdose rates as consumers accustomed to low quality heroin begin to encounter unpredictably higher purities following recent shifts in global trading patterns.

Retail heroin prices in Britain over the past 10 years have also been relatively constant. Just as there are variations in prevalence and modes of consumption from region to region, there are also variations in pricing. Prices are likely to be determined by proximity to ports of entry, importer/ distributor connections to countries of transit or origin, the availability of bulk supplies and the efficiency of the delivery system. The retail price of heroin in London in the early 1980s oscillated between £70 and £80 per gram (Lewis *et al.* 1985). After rising from £65 to £90 per gram between 1985 and 1986, prices steadied at £70–80 in early 1989. Even given a relative decline in purity since the early 1980s and a tendency over time for dealers to give shorter measures in 'bags' and 'wraps' (unweighed units), these figures suggest that, in London at least, the average retail price of heroin fell in real terms between 1980 and 1990 when set against inflation. Data for Glasgow suggest that prices were relatively stable over the past 5 years at £90–100 per gram (ISDD 1990). In Edinburgh, on the other hand, heroin cost as much as £140 per gram in 1990, despite the city's proximity to Glasgow. It may be possible to identify similar disparities between Liverpool and Manchester.

Distribution and delivery

Preble and Casey's six-level hierarchical outline of the New York delivery system (1969) remains relevant to European markets as a point of departure rather than as a blueprint. The following distribution categories have been elaborated from empirical observation by the author, and others, of markets in Britain and Italy and, to a lesser extent, France, Holland and Germany. They are broad approximations rather than rigid definitions:

1   importers and importer combinations;
2   distributors;
3   large-scale wholesalers;
4   small-scale wholesalers and apartment (house) dealers;
5   retail sales – street and appointment dealers, network suppliers and user-sellers;
6   end-users and street consumers.

Heroin distribution systems are composed of complex, articulated, multi-faceted series of layered networks, which individuals enter and exit according to means and circumstance. Despite restricted access to distribution levels, there are occasions when importers deliver directly to wholesalers, distributors, supply-house dealers, and ordinary consumers buy from wholesalers. The British national market is notably more flexible than some continental markets, which have higher barriers to entry constructed by organized crime groups that assert territorial control, exclude competitors and demand a share of all profits.

In countries like Italy there are fewer opportunities for individual initiative in the upper-echelons of the system, where criminal coalitions tend to dominate distribution. However, there is no universally applicable 'mafia' model of control in Italy or any other country. For instance, there is easy access to a range of quality and price arrangements in the strategically placed city of Verona where mafia-type groups have been all but marginalized by local traders (Arlacchi and Lewis 1990b).

Importers and bulk distributors

The development of distribution systems within Britain and Western Europe, as opposed to older-established trafficking enterprises directed at the United States, can be traced to the late 1960s and early 1970s. Heroin consumers, who were a minority within a wider pool of recreational drug users, lacked access to routine, wholesale connections. The common concern that bonded them at first found expression in long-distance 'ant-trafficking' (smuggling by individual consumers or groups in 'co-operative ventures') rather than in sustained large-scale business activity. With the perceived 'commercialization' of the drug subculture, such ventures tended to become less co-operative and more entrepreneurial. Without considerable investment, a sophisticated infrastructure and professional organization, international initiatives were increasingly risky, expensive and dangerous.

The arrival of bulk supplies of beige and brown South-west Asian heroin in Britain and Western Europe, between 1978 and 1980, coincided with the consolidation of a complex, high-turnover market. The size of consignments and the regularity of delivery clearly indicated that supply was being organized on a more systematic basis. Availability no longer depended upon individual journeys by ant-traffickers and user-dealers to Holland, India or Thailand. The acquisition and distribution of large quantities of heroin constituted a major business investment. Trading ceased to be simply a means: (1) to acquire heroin cheaply for personal consumption; or (2) to make a relatively modest living and subsidize future personal consumption through sales to other users.

In simple models of heroin distribution, the product commences its in-country trajectory as a high-quality kilo imported 'fresh off the boat'. It then passes by stages through the delivery system, where it is diluted to varying degrees, until it reaches the consumer as a retail unit. Some cities, like London, Amsterdam, Barcelona, Paris and Milan, function as points of importation, warehousing and brokerage. In zones where drugs transit in bulk quantities, there is frequent leakage on to local markets. In such situations, wholesale and retail prices may tend to be lower and purity proportionally higher because onward transportation and delivery costs are eliminated, and some of the intermediary stages within the distribution network are bypassed.

Bulk distributors and wholesalers are usually insulated from the street by three or four intermediary layers of distribution. In consequence, consumers and street-dealers know little about transactions at the apex of the system. Research information about the behaviour of distributors and wholesalers is normally the hardest to gather. Those involved in importation and bulk distribution are often full-time professional criminals, directly or indirectly connected in some parts of Europe to organized crime groups, which tends to make them both hostile and dangerous.

Bulk wholesalers

Importers, distributors, bulk wholesalers and house dealers (small-scale wholesalers), while performing different functions, all work in the wholesale sector. The bulk wholesaler bridges the middle ground between large-scale importer/distributors and low-level wholesalers and dealers. However, there are no hard and fast rules, particularly in cities where there is a high degree of mobility between layers of the market. Some independent distributors negotiate with apartment dealers. They may have narrower profit margins and no obligations to a wider organization, circumventing bulk wholesalers in order to sell directly to apartment dealers (small-scale wholesalers) or to dealers delivering directly to private elite circles. Bulk wholesalers may purchase:

1   directly from importers (or importer/producers who import semifinished goods (morphine or heroin base) and convert it to finished goods (heroin) as has occurred in Italy, France and Holland);
2   from distributors who have bought undiluted kilo units from importers or are acting on their behalf; or
3   travel to places of brokerage where they have their own contacts. One might normally expect wholesalers to purchase half-kilo to 100 g units and to sell diluted 100 to 30 g units to apartment dealers (small-scale wholesalers).

The kinds of individual involved at wholesale level can vary enormously from:

1   drug entrepreneurs, who in the past may have operated at retail level;
2   legitimate traders, who have developed sidelines as distributors or wholesalers (see also Dorn and South 1987);
3   predatory professional criminals, who have found a lucrative source of income in drugs.

On the whole, distributors and bulk wholesalers tend to be in their thirties and forties and have criminal records, while retail dealers and sellers, like most heroin consumers, are commonly in their twenties. Day-labourers working at street level as runners and look-outs can be in their teens.

Bulk suppliers are at their most vulnerable when taking or making deliveries. They are particularly exposed when:

1   collecting from large caches and fixed deposits;
2   transporting 30, 50 and 100 g units that cannot be justified as possession for personal use; and
3   making deliveries to customers.

Wholesalers may employ other individuals to perform such tasks. Evidence of wholesale delivery often emerges when there are seizures of gram and multi-gram quantities from house dealers and, for instance, empty 100 g bags containing traces of heroin are found on the same premises.

Small-scale wholesalers and apartment dealers

House (or apartment) dealers perform wholesale and retail functions. They buy 30 to 100 g units from bulk wholesalers that service a number of such enterprises and, on occasions, from upper-level distributors. They sell in 1–30 g lots to street, network and user-dealers, and directly to consumers. They are usually independent, although some may be franchised by criminal groups higher up the supply chain. Unlike network and street sellers, who can change location at will, the apartment dealer operates from a fixed base. This is normally an apartment or house, but may be a place of work or a bar. Places of legitimate business provide good cover in the sense that individuals can come and go without arousing suspicion and illicit income can be recycled through legitimate channels. The drawback of a fixed site is that once the location is identified by the police or hostile competitors, it becomes a relatively easy target. This also applies to fixed caches and stockpiles in isolated or rural hiding-places.

Ingold's description (1984) of Parisian apartment dealing in many ways resembles house dealing in cities like London. Ingold reports that assistants are frequently employed to answer the telephone, to find and select customers, and to collect and deliver money and/or drugs. They may be paid in money, drugs or both. The telephone, despite its vulnerability to interception, is an important instrument for receiving and relaying information. If the dealer is supplying both retailers and end-users, there is a possibility that the premises will become a place of consumption as well as distribution.

Dealers handling wholesale quantities of heroin also have to consider their own consumption. House dealers are normally users. If they fail to regulate personal use, they are liable to consume profits and stocks in the form of drugs. In consequence, they run the risk of exhausting their capital and resources, running into debt, going out of business and attracting the interest of enforcement by neglecting security. Even if they avoid prison, they may be left with a 5 g/day heroin habit that they can no longer afford. Hence, there is a constant tension between acquiring immediate satisfaction by consuming heroin as desired, and longer-term considerations of controlling levels of dependence in order to stay in business and guarantee future personal supplies.

Some transactions still may retain characteristics of personalized exchange and barter that were common to illicit drug markets prior to 1976. In such situations it is important that participants share a common history, and are known and accepted by their peers. They are normally members of restricted circles of heroin users of the kind found among small, discreet groups of recreational cannabis and cocaine users. They combine together to buy high-quality grams of heroin from wholesalers for their own consumption, and sometimes pool money as 'consumer co-operatives' to buy heroin in cities of importation or travel to producer nations in the manner of ant-traffickers.

Retail sales – street and appointment dealers, network suppliers and user-sellers

Most retail suppliers of heroin are consumers and, hence, user-dealers or user-sellers. The term 'dealer' is used to indicate an individual who supplies drugs for a cash return. The prospect of ready supplies of low-cost heroin is a prime motivation for entering the business. The lowest level of non-sedentary retail suppliers may be composed of:

1   appointment dealers;
2   street dealers;
3   network suppliers;
4   user-sellers; and
5   social suppliers.

Such categories serve to:

1   distinguish such suppliers from wholesale apartment dealers, who may also engage in retail supply;
2   emphasize that retail supply takes place in contexts other than the street or in purchases from apartment dealers;
3   encompass the fact that some retail suppliers cater for particular consumer networks by transferring the product to consumers on the supplier's premises, by visiting network members in their homes, or by appointment in a public or semi-public place.

Some consumers work as day-labourers in the market place. They switch service roles from day to day, fulfilling a variety of functions from testing, diluting and transporting heroin to selling, making introductions and keeping look-out. Such tasks are determined by what is most lucrative, least demeaning, least risky and least offensive to themselves (Johnson *et al.* 1985; Arlacchi and Lewis 1990b). The often chaotic ways that drugs are consigned publicly to end-users mean that arrests (effected as drugs change hands or soon afterwards) are a regular occurrence.

As relationships of mutual reciprocity, that were part of the earlier drug scene, broke down, transactions became progressively more detached and profit-oriented. As a result, drugs are less likely to be consumed and shared by buyer and seller in a group context. Many dealers do not wish to increase their vulnerability by employing their residence as a place of business or by dealing from a fixed location, nor do they want their customers, or their potential competitors, to know where they live. The appointment system partly developed for these reasons. It normally involves one supplier and six to 10 regular customers who keep in touch on a daily basis. Some cities have reported multi-personnel enterprises involving 200–300 transactions per day. Locations are alternated or changed, according to a pre-arranged plan, although purchasers are not informed of the site until close to the time of transaction. Telephones play an important role as do pagers, which are no longer esoteric New York-style accessories. They serve an important organizational function for some south London dealer networks.

The appointment system combines some of the characteristics of both apartment dealing and of street supply. Apartment dealing of wholesale and large retail units is common to most drug markets, as are sales in public locations where the product is dealt in minimal retail units by small-time dealers and user-sellers to consumers lacking better-placed connections. Appointment dealing constitutes a more discreet form of trading than random street sales. The rotation of locations avoids the risks entailed in a fixed site. Its drawback is that appointments normally take place in public or semi-public places. Hence, appointment dealing is:

1   planned in advance;
2   exposed, even though locations may be changed from day to day;
3   not suitable for prolonged negotiation or large-scale transactions that could involve the testing or weighing of the drug and, consequently, entails rapid retail trading;
4   subject to disruption by the inadvertent arrival of third parties, or through confusion about arrangements in the mind of the buyer or seller.

In spite of precautions, an employee or a telephone placed under surveillance can make the pre-arranged appointment as vulnerable as fixed-site dealing.

Some buyers try to establish relations with a regular dealer, who can be visited at home. Prior to this, an element of trust has to exist between buyer and seller. New clients normally have to be vouched for by regular customers. Apartment purchases are usually safer, cheaper and less subject to fraud than street purchases. Both dealer and customer have an investment in the continuity of the relationship. Apartment dealing is also less precarious than street dealing, although once an apartment has been identified by the police or the public, the dealer becomes more vulnerable than the street dealer, who, if he is lucky, can disappear without trace.

On the street itself, points of refurbishment and sale tend to be in continual flux. News travels fast on illicit consumer networks. In large markets some open-air, multi-product, retail enterprises are organized in a very sophisticated fashion. Appointment dealers frequently change distribution points around the city on a day-to-day basis to avoid police surveillance. Runners, look-outs and messengers, paid in money, drugs or both, are systematically co-ordinated. Deliveries may be made by car, motor cycle or public transport. In large retail enterprises, supplies are purchased directly from bulk wholesalers, circumventing apartment dealers who probably could not fulfil demand on a daily basis.

'Historic' public dealing venues such as Piccadilly in central London, the Dam in Amsterdam, the Zoo in Berlin and the Parco Lambro in Milan tend to be places where:

1   casual users or young initiates, unfamiliar with the market, come to buy;

2   old-style street survivors congregate, partly to stay in touch and, partly, in the hope of obtaining drugs or cash by interposing themselves between retail dealers and potential customers; and

3   regular consumers, whose usual points of supply have been lost or terminated, seek a temporary substitute. Quality is usually lower, prices higher, weights shorter, and theft and fraud more frequent in such a context. 'Birds of passage', surviving on the social fringes of a host country, are able to work as suppliers in such high-profile locations because of their very transience. They are vulnerable as single individuals but, because of their impermanence, the dealing in which they engage is less subject to systematic police and monopolistic criminal pressure.

The vulnerability of heroin market participants, and the ability of violent criminals to intimidate them, is enhanced by:

1   criminal domination of some illicit markets;

2   the physical dependence of addicts and their need to expose themselves in search of both drugs and money;

3   the limited sources of alternative supply;

4   the reputation and capacity of criminal entrepreneurs for carrying out their threats; and

5   the illegality of much addict behaviour and consequent lack of recourse to the police. Some consumers argue that levels of violence may be directly proportional to the availability of heroin. The more heroin that is available, the less theft, conflict and violence occurs at street level. When there is a

heroin shortage incidents of fraud and theft increase. Frustrated demand, in other words, appears to be a major cause of violence.

The violence that occurs usually:

1 happens between users;
2 is imposed on users by other predatory users or as part of a punitive mechanism within the distribution system; or
3 is imposed by outsiders attached to criminal and, sometimes, law enforcement bodies.

The resilience and adaptability of the heroin delivery systems described above, in the face of sustained enforcement pressure, raises questions as to the usefulness of contemporary prohibitionist models of control. It is possible that a formally regulated and taxed market might lead to a reduction in the drug-related harm, revenue-raising crime and violence that are associated with illicit heroin economies. The fact that such a taboo subject is now a matter for lively debate suggests that in Europe, if not the United States, the regulation of drug markets is being seen as a practical policy issue rather than as just one more business opportunity for moral entrepreneurs.

References

Arlacchi, P. and Lewis, R. (1987). Analisi del mercato delle droghe e sua influenza ai fini delta determinazione delta categoria giuridica delta modica quantita. Ministero di Grazia e Giustizia, Rome.

Arlacchi, P. and Lewis, R. (1990a). Droga e criminalita a Bologna. *Micromega*, 4, 183–221.

Arlacchi, P. and Lewis, R. (1990b). *Imprenditorialita illecita e droga – il mercato dell' eroina a Verona*. Il Mulino, Bologna.

de Alarcon, R. (1973). Lessons from the recent British drug outbreak. Proceedings of the Anglo-American conference on drug abuse. Royal Society of Medicine, London.

Dorn, N. and South, N. (1987). Some issues in the development of drug markets and law enforcement. Working paper, workshop on drugs, 22–23 October. Commission of the European Communities, Luxembourg.

Fraser, A. and George, M. (1988). Changing trends in drug use, an initial follow-up of a local heroin-using community. *British Journal of Addiction*, 83, 655–63.

Haw, S. (1985). Drug problems in Greater Glasgow. Standing conference on drug abuse, Glasgow.

Haw, S. and Liddell, D. (1989). Drug problems in Edinburgh district. Standing conference on drug abuse, London.

Ingold, R. (1984). La dependance economique chez les heroinomanes. *Revue Internationale de Police Criminelle*, 391, 208–13, ottobre.

INCB (1989). Report of the International Narcotics Control Board. United Nations, New York.

ISDD (1990). Drug misuse in Britain. National audit of drug misuse statistics. Institute for the Study of Drug Dependence, London.

Johnson, B. D., Goldstein, P. J. and Preble, E. (1985). *Taking care of business – the economics of crime by heroin abusers.* Lexington Books, Lexington, MA.

Lewis, R., Hartnoll, R., Bryer, S., Daviaid, E. and Mitcheson, M. (1985). Scoring smack – the illicit heroin market in London, 1980–1983. *British Journal of Addiction*, 80, 281–90.

Mott, J. and Rathod, N. H. (1976). Heroin use and delinquency in a new town. *British Journal of Psychiatry*, 128, 428–35.

Parker, H., Bakx, K. and Newcombe, R. (1986). Drug misuse in Wirral, a study of 1800 problem drug users known to official agencies. The first report. University of Liverpool, Liverpool.

Pearson, G., Gilman, M. and McIver, S. (1987). Young people and heroin, examination of heroin use in the north of England. Gower Health Education Council, Aldershot.

Power, R. (1990). Patterns of drug use and some recent research developments in Britain. In *Epidemiologic trends in drug abuse* (ed. N. Kozel), Vol. II, pp. 83–104. Proceedings. National Institute on Drug Abuse, Rockville, MD.

Preble, E. and Casey, J. J. (1969). Taking care of business, the heroin user's life on the street. *International Journal of the Addictions*, 4, 1–24.

Redlinger, L. J. (1974). Marketing and distributing heroin. *Journal of Psychedelic Drugs*, 1, 331–53.

Chapter 9

Drug epidemics in space and time

Local diversity, subcultures and social exclusion

Geoffrey Pearson and Mark Gilman

The drug-related problems which have visited many parts of Europe and North America in the second half of the twentieth century are not evenly distributed in space and time. Rather, they come in the form of epidemics which result in wide variations between different regions and localities in terms of the form and level of difficulty experienced, the types of drugs involved, the social characteristics of drug users, and the ways in which drugs are consumed.

Drug habits and preferences are established and maintained through human contact, and it is for this reason that the 'contagious disease' model of drug transmission proposed by Patrick Hughes and his colleague seems fundamentally important in understanding drug epidemics (Hughes and Crawford, 1972). Of course, the notion of human 'contagion' does not mean that the spread of drug habits and preferences is simply a passive biological process of 'contagion' or 'infection'. Rather, decisions whether or not to experiment with drugs of different kinds, or whether to continue using them and in what ways, are shaped both by the various social meanings which attach to drugs, and also whether or not their psycho-pharmacological properties cohere with people's lifestyle and self-image. That it to say, these are active socio-cultural and socio-economic exchanges between different sets of drug users and non-users, experimental users and committed users, past-users, part-timers and quitters – lines of interaction along which drug habits flow and which can either initiate, sustain or terminate drugs epidemics.

The aim of this chapter is to review what is known about these kinds of local and regional variations, the ways in which spatial and demographic diversity reflects subcultural preferences, and the fact that the most serious drug-related problems typically come to be associated with social exclusion. Overall, the aim will be both one of description and to provide a theoretical and conceptual framework for understanding these processes. The main focus will be the British experience – specifically the heroin epidemic which had its onset in the early-to-mid-1980s, and which continues to be the defining problem in many parts of Britain – although the chapter will also draw upon a wider body of research evidence, particularly from the USA. Our underlying argument will be that local and regional diversity of drug-related problems has strategic importance for policy analysis and service development. In a concluding section we will draw from US experience to indicate what can be learned from monitoring drug epidemics over time.

Heroin diversity in the North of England: the initial impact of the 1980s epidemic

Our interest in the social and geographical diversity of drug misuse had first arisen in the context of research for the Health Education Council on the emerging heroin epidemic in the North of England during the mid-1980s (Pearson et al., 1985). This region was one of the major sites of the 1980s heroin epidemic, and a brief sketch of its initial impact will offer some illustrative empirical detail of the forms of diversity with which the analysis must contend.

Heroin made an abrupt entrance in the North of England at some point in the early 1980s when the drug became available in cheap and plentiful supply – predominantly through new trade routes from the 'Golden Crescent' of South West Asia (Iran, Afghanistan, Pakistan) as opposed to importation from the opium-fields of the 'Golden Triangle' of South East Asia. This major geo-political shift in opium production and heroin trafficking was certainly felt elsewhere in Britain, including London where there was already a well-established subculture of heroin injecting (Burr, 1987; Lewis et al., 1985). One crucial difference where the North of England was concerned is that in the course of the 1980s heroin misuse became a significant social problem in many towns and cities where, unlike London, it had been previously quite unknown. The earlier and much less extensive heroin epidemic which had peaked in the late 1960s, described in detail by Stimson and Oppenheimer (1982), made very little impact outside of London. Equally important is that the new 'brown' heroin which became available in the 1980s was in smokable form and that the early 1980s epidemic in the North of England was indelibly associated with the novel practice of 'chasing the dragon' (Parker et al., 1988; Pearson et al., 1985; Pearson, 1987a).

Against these broadly uniform developments, a sharp geographical division was clearly observable in the North of England between those sub-regions which were situated either to the East or West of the Pennine range of hills – the so-called 'backbone' of England. Heroin misuse spread much more rapidly in the West than in the East, and not only in the major urban conurbations of Manchester and Liverpool, but also in many of the small towns in the Lancashire 'cotton belt' of the western Pennines. Heroin use was certainly not unknown in the Yorkshire towns and cities to the East, where just as in the West there were pre-existing small subcultures of opiate adepts, but it did not assume the rapid wildfire growth which was evident in many parts of Manchester, Merseyside and the smaller Lancashire towns

(Pearson *et al.*, 1985). If this East–West divide was a dominant aspect of the geographical diversity of heroin use at an early point of the epidemic in the mid-1980s, it has not remained so. Already in the early 1990s there was evidence of a sharp increase of new heroin users in the city of Bradford and elsewhere in Yorkshire (Pearson and Patel, 1998). Subsequently, the heroin outbreaks of the late 1990s charted by Parker, Bury and Egginton (1998) have changed the map in this and many other regions of England. Drug epidemics, by their very nature, do not stand still.

Broad geographical variations such as the East–West Pennine divide in the 1980s result from the drug dissemination processes known as 'macro-diffusion'. These are amply described by Hunt and Chambers (1976) in their detailed study of the American heroin epidemic between 1965 and 1975, a study which mapped the spread of heroin availability and heroin use across the vast continental landmass of the USA. Heroin use had already been an established feature of the life of several major US cities prior to the heroin epidemics of the late 1960s. The earliest postwar heroin epidemic in Chicago had peaked in 1949 (Hughes *et al.*, 1972). In New York, on the other hand, although heroin and opium use were already known in the 1920s and 1930s, it was not until the mid-to-late 1950s that it began to emerge as a major social difficulty (Courtwright *et al.*, 1989; Preble and Casey, 1969). From the mid-1960s onwards, however, as Hunt and Chambers demonstrated in impressive detail, heroin misuse began to spread outwards from those cities with an already-existing problem – not by any means in a uniform manner, but in a way which exhibited numerous local and regional variations. The factors which determined how this dispersal of heroin's availability and the creation of potential markets unfolded were largely matters of geographical distance, the ease or difficulty of transport routes, difficult terrain, patterns of human migration, etc. Moreover, this epidemic process in the late 1960s and early 1970s would establish a social and geographical pattern of heroin misuse which was still found to be a major influence on patterns of heroin use in the USA twenty-five years later (Boyum and Rochelau, 1994).

In a much smaller country such as England, a late-1960s study by De Alarcon (1969) had shown how a hit-and-miss friendship network could assist in the 'macro-diffusion' of heroin use and availability from London so as to produce a mini-epidemic of heroin misuse in the south coast towns of Brighton and Worthing (see description in Chapter 5, this volume). This offers a useful reminder of how broad structures of 'macro-diffusion' between regions, towns and cities can be assisted or inhibited by the much more local and circumstantial patterns of 'micro-diffusion' among friends, neighbours and acquaintances. Whatever the precise mechanism – whether an informal friendship network, the movement of migrant workers who might introduce a new drug habit into the area in which they settle, or a determined criminal conspiracy to establish a new distribution system and to extend the market for an illicit drug – it is macro-diffusion processes which underpin variations between cities and regions in terms of drug availability and consequently of the possibility for an illicit drug subculture to take root. Nevertheless, local circumstance and pre-existing subcultural preferences and lifestyles are by no means passive in these regards, and it is to these that we now turn.

Smokers, snorters and injectors: local and regional variations

In contrast to the grand East–West Pennines divide, a second aspect of geographical diversity was to be found *within* those towns and cities which developed a heroin problem in the 1980s. These 'urban clustering' effects will be discussed in more detail at a later point. Suffice to say that highly localised variations in how drug-related problems manifest themselves have enormous implications for practical interventions – whether in terms of the use of outreach to better understand nuanced variations 'on the ground', the siting and orientation of service delivery, or local enforcement tactics.

One further notable aspect of local and regional diversity concerned the route of administration of the drug – principally whether it was injected or smoked. This might seem to be a more idiosyncratic matter, but initial observations in the 1980s indicated distinguishable patterns of geographical variation. As already indicated, the upsurge of heroin use in the 1980s was largely associated with the practice of 'chasing the dragon', and the rapid spread of the habit was facilitated by the fact that it did not involve novice users transgressing the formidable cultural taboo of self-injection. There were some areas of the North of England, however, where the novel heroin epidemic was immediately associated with self-injection.

Given that the upsurge in heroin use emerged prior to any widespread recognition of the risks of HIV infection through sharing injecting equipment, this was not an immediate consideration either for drug users or service providers. When the Department of Health did begin to collect information on injecting patterns, as part of the notification system for the Addicts Index, this revealed some sharp regional and local disparities (Pearson and Gilman, 1994, pp. 112–15). For example, in 1988 the reported rate of injecting varied from as low as 39 per cent in the Mersey Regional Health Authority and 59 per cent in the North Western region – both major sites of the new heroin epidemic – as against 80 per cent in Oxford, Yorkshire and East Anglia. Within the Mersey region itself, moreover, there were complex variations between different District Health Authorities – as low as 30 per cent in the Wirral peninsula, as against 63 per cent in nearby Macclesfield (ibid., Table 8.3). What might have determined these local variations?

The immediate impression was that these local variations in drug-using practices were largely a result of differences in pre-existing drug cultures within different localities and regions. Primarily, whether any form of intravenous drug-using culture had existed prior to the arrival of the 'new' heroin, organised largely around the use of amphetamines together with various forms of polydrug use (Pearson *et al.*, 1985). Where amphetamine sulphate had previously been injected, for example, with the arrival of heroin this pre-existing attitude towards 'powder' drugs would be applied to the new drug. Where amphetamine powder might have been sniffed or snorted, 'chasing' seemed more likely to emerge as the preferred method. Relatively high injection rates in the town of Macclesfield, for example, reflected the existence of a small but persistent injecting drug subculture since the 1970s. Whereas in the Wirral peninsula, which was one of the major sites of the 'chasing' phenomenon, heroin became so widely available and so widely used that many of the 'new' users had no prior contact with or knowledge of injecting drug practices.

The ways in which drugs are consumed – in this case either smoked or injected – is but one aspect of how novice users are socialised into an existing drug culture, which like any other culture will combine its own set of meanings, recipes for action and practices. Because drug use and drug users' preferences are not simply a question of pharmacology, but also cultural meaning and fashion (Pearson, 1992). Some illustrations of these combinations of pharmacology and fashion will be offered in the next section.

Subcultural styles and meanings: pharmacology and fashion

The fact that heroin had been a quite unknown drug in many parts of the North of England prior to its sudden availability in the early 1980s did not mean that other forms of drug use – predominantly cannabis, but also hallucinogens such as LSD, amphetamines and various stimulant pills – were also unknown. Local drug cultures were also associated with other aspects of popular culture such as the 1970s 'Northern Soul' music scene, with its own pattern of recreational drug use which had been largely focused on amphetamines (Wilson, 1999). These provided the basis from which young people in different localities responded to the arrival of heroin – either in terms of acceptance or rejection – since already-existing drug subcultures could prove to be either receptive or resistant to the novel appearance of heroin in the early 1980s. These interactions could sometimes be quite idiosyncratic.

In one locality, for example, there was an established preference among young people for a recreational lifestyle organised around relaxing to music, with the accompaniment of cannabis smoking and the more occasional use of 'magic mushrooms'. Some had tried heroin when it first became available, but did not like the drug which they described as 'too heavy a stone', and which was incompatible with their established recreational pursuits. Elsewhere, in a small Lancashire town, members of a local Skinhead youth culture in the early 1980s had formed a cultural opposition towards cannabis and hallucinogens because of the association, as they saw it, between these drugs and 'hippies' with their attachment to outmoded fashions such as long hair and flared trousers. Heroin, for them, was a culturally attractive drug since it was overtly rejected by the hippie generation, and had been embraced by members of the Skinhead gang as a more 'manly' drug, the use of which expressed their 'hardness' and daring. In this way their response was reminiscent of Feldman's description of the appeal of heroin to tough street-fighting gangs in New York's lower East Side during the 1960s heroin epidemic in the United States (Feldman, 1968).

The cultural and subcultural dimensions of drug preferences, and how these adhere to wider aspects of popular culture have been analysed by writers such as Paul Willis (1978) and Angela Burr (1984) – discussing, respectively, hippie attitudes towards 'soft' and 'hard' drugs, and the nihilistic attraction of barbiturates amidst the 'ideologies of despair' embraced by Punk and Skinhead youth cultures (see Chapter 6, this volume). Our point here is that these subcultural preferences can also have a distinctively local flavour – whether in terms of the types of drugs used, or how they are used.

The subcultural 'how' of drug use is not solely a matter of the route of administration – smoked, injected, swallowed, inhaled – although this is not unimportant. It can also involve the ambience within which drugs are consumed, in what dosage levels, with what frequency, etc. For some drugs these matters are determined by pharmacology – too high or too frequent a dose leads to overdose – for others it is a question of how levels and forms of use are assimilated to different lifestyles.

One illustrative study of subcultural variations in terms of how the same drug might be used is offered by Munoz and Davis (1969) in their account of the Haight Ashbury drug scene in late 1960s San Francisco. They describe two opposed approaches towards the use of LSD: the 'true' hippies or 'Heads' on the one side who surrounded LSD use with various rituals and used the drug in a contemplative if not quasi-religious way; as against the 'Freaks' who were accused by the 'true' believers of merely 'tripping out' on LSD, and who were also more likely to inject methedrine. This contrast between a cool, contemplative use of LSD and the more libidinal, hedonistic aim of getting 'bombed out' is not dissimilar to the contrasting ways in which MDMA (Ecstasy) is currently used in the USA and Britain. In North America MDMA is more likely to be used in a contemplative setting and only on a very occasional basis, whereas in Britain it is a drug often used regularly at weekends, sometimes involving binge use, and invariably in the context of the 'rave' culture of all-night high-velocity music (Beck and Rosenbaum, 1994; Hammersley et al., 1999; Pearson et al., 1991).

One final example of the diverse patterns of drug use which gathered around the 1980s heroin epidemic in the North of England concerns neither the subcultural meanings of drugs, nor the route of administration – but quite simply a persistent pharmacological preference within a local drug culture. Prior to the onset of the heroin epidemic in some parts of North

West England there had been an established preference for Diconal among already existing, albeit small, communities of injecting opiate users. Diconal was, and indeed still is, a pharmaceutical formulation in tablet form which contained a mixture of the opioid dipipanone and cyclizine which has anti-emetic properties. Following the re-classification of Diconal in 1984, it became much more difficult to obtain by medical prescription. However, some of these local drug cultures maintained a preference for Diconal in spite of the increasingly widespread availability of 'street' heroin. Some users of this drug maintained that it had distinctive and valued psycho-pharmacological effects – sometimes known as the 'Diconal freezes' – including hallucino-genic episodes. As already indicated, one of the constituents of Diconal is the anti-emetic cyclizine, and there is a small but scattered literature on the misuse of cyclizine where it is reported that users experienced hallucinations of various kinds (Gilman et al., 1990). With the interruption of the supply of Diconal, 'street alchemists' within these drug-using communities set about attempting to re-constitute its effects – eventually landing upon a combina-tion of methadone, which could be obtained by prescription, and travel sickness preparations which contained cyclizine and could be bought as over-the-counter medicines at pharmacy outlets. Such was the fashion for this 'do-it-yourself' Diconal that in one Lancashire town pharmacists banned the sale of cyclizine – with the effect that in the late 1980s an illicit trade in the drug was established, with cyclizine tablets which would normally have cost a few pence changing hands for £2.50 at the street-level of this market (Gilman, 1988; Gilman et al., 1990).

We can therefore see how pharmacology and fashion are variously intertwined in different drug subcultures. It is important to recognise that sometimes these subcultures embrace ideologies of reckless and potentially self-destructive drug consumption. At other times, they involve rules and meanings which regulate and control patterns of drug consumption, and set limits to excessive or compulsive use (Zinberg, 1984). Indeed, we can point to certain patterns of established recreational drug use which involve cultures of opposition towards the use of certain drugs such as heroin or crack-cocaine (Pearson, 2001). These are illicit drug cultures, in other words, which are relatively benign and which give no support to 'gateway' theories of drug escalation – whereby the use of one illicit drug supposedly projects the user onto an inevitable career of deepening drug involvement. But there are also circumstances in which local communities can be highly susceptible to escalat-ing dangers and drug-related problems, and it is to these that we now turn.

Vulnerable communities: 'urban clustering' and social exclusion

One of the most consistent findings of research on the social and spatial dimensions of drug misuse is for the most serious aspects of drug-related difficulty to be densely concentrated in the poorest neighbourhoods which also experience other multiple social problems such as housing deprivation, mass unemployment, high levels of crime and the fear of crime. A trend first noted in the USA, it was to be amply confirmed in the context of the 1980s British heroin epidemic and its legacy. In this section we will briefly review the evidence, and then offer a policy-relevant model aimed at understanding the various dimensions of these 'urban clustering' effects.

A systematic social scientific approach to the urban ecology of social problems had been first developed by the Chicago School of Sociology in the 1920s and 1930s in a programme of research which was to prove vastly influential. Studies such as those by Shaw and McKay (1942) on juvenile delinquency, together with that by Faris and Dunham (1939) on mental disorder, pointed to a dense concentration of these social difficulties in the poor areas of what we would now call Chicago's 'inner city'. The area was characterised by cheap rented accommodation, many local residents were recently arrived migrant workers, and it also experienced high levels of tuberculosis and suicide. In addition, as indicated by an often neglected study of opium addiction by Bingham Dai (1937), this, too, was densely concentrated in Chicago's poor inner-urban zone and scarcely encountered in the city's outskirts and suburbs.

In bald terms, the Chicago School's pioneering work set the pattern for subsequent North American research on the social and geographical spread of drug misuse within cities. In their 1950s New York study of narcotics and delinquency, Chein et al. (1964) found these to be concentrated in areas of socio-economic disadvantage, while ethnographic research would show how this cohered with the lifestyles and local economies of New York's ghetto neighbourhoods (Feldman, 1968; Preble and Casey, 1969). In Chicago, employing a combination of ethnographic and epidemiological methods to provide a detailed mapping of local heroin outbreaks between 1967 and 1971, Patrick Hughes and his colleagues found that 'the largest outbreaks occurred in economically disadvantaged communities' (Hughes, 1977, p. 75; Hughes and Crawford, 1972). Research of a different kind in Baltimore, involving an area analysis of ecological correlations, indicated the same clustering effect of levels of drug misuse, crime and multiple deprivation (Nurco, 1972; Nurco et al., 1984). Ethnographic fieldwork on heroin-related crime in East and Central Harlem and on the crack-cocaine epidemic in this and other parts of New York City, combining research on patterns of drug misuse and the economic structure of local drug markets, provided further evidence of how in the 1980s and 1990s these problems remained embedded in the same circumstances of urban decay and social exclusion (Johnson et al., 1985; Williams, 1989; Bourgois, 1995; Maher, 1997).

In the wake of the 1980s heroin epidemic, this pattern of 'urban clustering' would reproduce itself in many parts of Britain whereby the most dense concentrations of drug-related difficulty would take root in the poorest neighbourhoods and housing estates which were already experiencing high levels of unemployment and social deprivation. In an early phase of the heroin epidemic in Glasgow, Haw (1985, p. 53) found that 'the majority of identified opiate users come from the poorest areas of the city', with other early indications of this same trend coming from our own fieldwork in a number of areas of the North of England (Pearson et al., 1985). In a study of national trends, Peck and Plant (1986) also pointed to a correlation between the sharp rise in unemployment in the early 1980s and increasing levels of problematic drug misuse. It was, however, at a local level that these developments were most pronounced, and other local studies using different methodologies confirmed the socio-economic and spatial concentration of the difficulty. The most important of these undoubtedly was the major research undertaking on the Wirral peninsula in Merseyside, which through a combination of methods – the analysis of agency records, field studies and snowballing chain-referral techniques – established high correlations between local prevalence levels of heroin misuse and a variety of social deprivation indicators (Parker et al., 1988. See Chapter 7, this volume). Other studies which confirmed this picture included that of Class A drug users in Nottingham (Giggs et al., 1989), the geo-demographic analysis of patients attending a drug dependency clinic in Liverpool (Fazey et al., 1990), together with fieldwork and survey analysis of heroin and cocaine use in different parts of south London (Burr, 1987; Mirza et al., 1991; Pearson et al., 1993).

The mechanisms involved in bringing together these 'urban clustering' effects are undoubtedly complex, and a variety of influences are at work (Pearson and Gilman, 1994; Pearson, 1987b, 1995). From a practical point of view, the important issue is that the most serious drug-related problems take root in those neighbourhoods which are already experiencing a multitude of social difficulties. Since its origins in the mid-1980s, for example, the British Crime Survey (BCS) has shown that there is a distinct tendency for the highest levels of criminal victimisation and the 'fear of crime' phenomenon also to be found in our poorest neighbourhoods (Hough and Mayhew, 1985). On a wider European canvas, a study of the most socially disadvantaged housing estates in northern Europe has also found that problems of crime and drug misuse were often interwoven among multiple social difficulties (Power, 1997).

Indeed, perhaps the most crucial mechanism which brings together these multiple problems is the working of the housing market. Research on the 'criminal careers' of residential neighbourhoods has for some time offered useful insights into the ways in which the housing market can shape variations in the crime rate (Bottoms and Wiles, 1986; Bottoms et al., 1989). Where a so-called 'problem estate' begins to attract a reputation for various kinds of notoriety, only those with the most urgent housing need will be prepared to accept a tenancy (Reynolds, 1986). These will include those who are homeless or near-homeless, single-parent households and women escaping from domestic violence, together with other groups with limited options in the housing market such as the elderly poor. One characteristic which problem drug users share with these other groups is that they, too, will often be marginal to the housing market. So that these social and economic forces conspire to gather together in these already embattled neighbourhoods a variety of otherwise unrelated social and personal difficulties.

Where problem drug users do settle in neighbourhoods such as these – whether through regular tenancies, emergency short-term housing schemes, or squatting in empty dwellings – one further consequence is that the likely availability of drugs within the locality will be increased. This set of circumstances thereby provides the fertile ground upon which local drug epidemics can develop, given that it is local friendship networks which spread drug habits within a neighbourhood (cf. Hughes and Crawford, 1972; Pearson, 1987a). It is also possible that local drug habits spread more quickly and with more serious consequences in areas of social deprivation. As Zinberg's (1984) work has shown, the possibilities for controlled intoxicant use are considerably enhanced when a person has other valued life commitments – such as employment – which cannot be reconciled with heavy drug consumption. Where such claims are absent, it is more likely that drug experimentation will be more quickly consolidated into a regular habit, and that habitual drug use will assume a compulsive and potentially self-destructive form.

One further way in which certain patterns of drug misuse cohere with the lifestyles of those who suffer social exclusion is well documented in the tradition of social research into the development of deviant subcultures and delinquency (Pearson, 1994). Where young people experience inequality in terms of educational and employment opportunities, alternative systems of status, achievement and rewards come to be established. These might involve prowess in fighting or thieving, and as ethnographic research vividly demonstrates in the context of both the heroin and crack-cocaine epidemics in the USA, involvement in drug subcultures can offer another route to local status in deprived neighbourhoods (Preble and Casey, 1969; Feldman, 1968; Bourgois, 1995).

Most importantly, this research showed that although drug misuse is often characterised as a form of 'escapism' and 'retreatism', the daily routines of the street addict involve an extremely hectic lifestyle known in American drug slang as 'taking care of business' (Preble and Casey, 1969; Johnson et al., 1985). This active lifestyle came to many parts of Britain in the wake of the 1980s heroin epidemic whereby in order to maintain a drug habit, the user must engage in 'a hectic flurry of hustles and economic exchanges, requiring considerable resourcefulness, economic dexterity and entrepreneurial skill and commitment' (Gilman and Pearson, 1991, p. 95). Thus, 'when not searching for money or drugs to start the day, the heroin user was trying to avoid the police, looking for a safe place to "get off", searching again for money and the next bag, in an endless cycle of activity . . . a job of work, a kind of work, moreover, which was seven days a week with no rest days' (ibid., p. 95). Commitment to this hectic lifestyle might even, then, offer a kind of solution to the problem of unemployment and idleness, albeit one which was potentially destructive. Even so, an unsentimental attitude will also recognise that tangible monetary gains also exist through involvement in the retail drug trade, thereby further cementing the relationships between drugs and deprivation (Reuter et al., 1990; Bourgois, 1995). As Williams and Kornblum (1985, p. 59) describe it in their study of young people growing up in poverty-stricken neighbourhoods, 'the time honoured drive to "get ahead" explains why the underground economy tends to flourish in direct proportion to decreases in regular employment opportunities and public spending for education, employment, and training'.

Drug misuse is not restricted to the poor and those who suffer from other forms of social exclusion, of course, and is found to some degree in all sections of society. Nevertheless, as outlined above, research in the USA, Britain and other parts of Europe has consistently pointed to the ways in which the most serious drug problems are concentrated in the poorest neighbourhoods. Moreover, as the British heroin epidemic of the 1980s brutally demonstrated at a time of very high levels of youth unemployment, heroin misuse can spread with wildfire rapidity in vulnerable communities under circumstances such as these.

The accumulated evidence on the relationships between drug misuse and social exclusion was systematically reviewed in the report on *Drug Misuse and the Environment* by the UK Government's Advisory Council on the Misuse of Drugs. Its conclusion was emphatic:

> We thus assert without any of the familiar hedging with 'on the one hand but on the other', that on strong balance of probability deprivation is today in Britain likely often to make a significant causal contribution to the cause, complication and intractability of damaging kinds of drug misuse . . . We want now and in the future to see deprivation given its full and proper place in all considerations of drug prevention policy, held in that policy consciousness, and not let slip from sight.
>
> (ACMD, 1998, pp. 113, 115)

It would no doubt be an interesting study in the history of ideas as to how the immediately obvious connection in the mid-1980s between drugs and deprivation evidenced by countless local heroin epidemics on housing estates in cities such as Manchester, Liverpool, Glasgow, Edinburgh and inner-London remained ignored and denied in public policy, as social exclusion and the social consequences of high unemployment were marginalised by successive Conservative administrations throughout the 1980s and early 1990s. The Advisory Council's recognition that drug-related problems are closely intertwined with social deprivation is thus a landmark in British social policy, and is now also formally enshrined in the UK government's ten-year drug strategy announced in 1998 (President of the Council, 1998). On one level, this involves the strategic objective to protect communities from drug-related anti-social nuisance and criminal behaviour. Also, in what undoubtedly involves a major challenge, to conceive of services for problem drug users as more than 'coming off' drugs and to position them within wider socio-economic programmes and systems of social reintegration in terms of employment, job training, housing support and urban regeneration.

Monitoring drug epidemics: learning from the North American experience

Local and regional variations in levels and patterns of drug use are therefore one of the defining characteristics of the nature of drug-related problems. Indeed, one might almost say that it is wrong to think of the problem of drug misuse as a national problem; rather, it is better conceived of as a series of loosely articulated local and regional difficulties, each with its own differences in terms of form and content. Moreover, although the evidence base is much weaker for drug enforcement and the supply side, it seems likely that drug markets and drug availability exhibit similar local and regional variations (Bennett, 2000; Pearson and Hobbs, 2001).

In this section, the weakness of the research and evidence base in these regards in Britain will be addressed, together with some discussion of how drug epidemics might be monitored and mapped, including discussion of what can be learned from one such drug monitoring programme in the USA. Because although the broad geographical patterning of the early 1980s heroin epidemic in the North of England seemed quite straightforward, we do not have any systematic evidence of how such spatial variations in drug misuse have subsequently developed in modern Britain.

What evidence we do have is at best sketchy. The 'four town' Home Office survey of the early 1990s suggested considerable variations between the different sites – Glasgow and the London Borough of Lewisham scoring higher than Nottingham and Bradford – but this offered only a very general impression of self-reported illicit drug use, largely cannabis use, with only very small numbers of problematic heroin or cocaine users captured in the survey sample (Leitner *et al.*, 1993). We know from more localised research that substantial numbers of problem drug users were to be found in both Glasgow and Lewisham (Haw, 1985; McKeganey and Barnard, 1992; Mirza *et al.*, 1991; Pearson *et al.*, 1993; Taylor, 1993, 1998), but the 'four town' study offered only a distant reflection of this. Nor was it able to register the rapid increase in heroin use which was already under way in Bradford and other parts of West Yorkshire in the early 1990s (Pearson and Patel, 1998).

Attempts have also been made to trace regional patterns using self-report data from the British Crime Survey (BCS), although again very small proportions of problematic drug users are involved and these attempts largely encompass the use of cannabis and 'dance drugs' (Ramsay and Percy, 1996, pp. 40, 92; Ramsay and Spiller, 1997, pp. 32–3; Ramsay and Partridge, 1999, p. 74). Even so, year-on-year comparisons within some regions have implied such volatile changes as to suggest that these are the consequence of sampling and design factors within the BCS. Indeed, British surveys of illicit drug use are more generally under-powered in terms of sample size, and can offer few meaningful comparisons either between regions or across time (Gore, 1999). We therefore know very little about the comparative regional penetration of heroin and cocaine in Britain in the 1990s, although on the available evidence it seems highly likely that there might be both regional and other important forms of socio-demographic and/or localised variation.

In the USA, with its much longer history of problematic drug misuse, there is also a consolidated experience of different means of mapping and monitoring drug epidemics (Hughes and Rieche, 1995). One promising line of development for surveying regional variations in problematic drug use is offered by the US programme of urine-analysis among samples of arrestees held in police custody (NIJ, 1998). A limited pilot study in a small number of areas in England has already shown its potential, indicating marked variations in positive tests for selected drugs between some of these sites (Bennett, 1998, p. 16; 2000, p. 42).

Formerly known as Drug Use Forecasting (DUF), this urine-testing programme which now covers 23 sites across the USA has recently been re-fashioned and re-named the Arrestee Drug Abuse Monitoring (ADAM) programme. Initiated in the mid-1980s, the DUF/ADAM programme has been able to offer multiple insights into shifting patterns of drug misuse among this high-risk group of arrestees. The main concern in the USA in this period has been cocaine misuse, and DUF/ADAM has been able to track how the crack-cocaine epidemic has begun to wane in some US cities, with sharp falls in the 1990s in nine of the dozen sites participating in the late 1980s DUF programme (cf. NIJ, 1989, 1997, 1998). Even so, among 23 ADAM sites in 1997, in only 4 sites did fewer than 25 per cent of males test positive for cocaine, whereas in 9 sites 40–60 per cent tested positive (NIJ, 1998).

Detailed secondary analysis of the waning US cocaine epidemic further highlights the potential of the DUF/ADAM programme – both as a tool for epidemiological research and as a policy instrument – showing substantial variations between different cities in the trajectory of local cocaine epidemics, with specific age-cohort effects (Golub and Johnson, 1994, 1997). Violent crime has also begun to fall in cities where the cocaine epidemic is receding (Baumer et al., 1999). In New York, for example, since the early 1990s younger people have seen the damage done by crack-cocaine and have begun to reject it; although high levels of positive tests are still found among older, already addicted, cohorts. Ethnographic work conducted by the same research team in New York confirms the qualitative features of these changes, whereby African-American and Latino youths in ghetto districts are turning away from crack-cocaine towards marijuana, often smoked in hollowed-out 'Blunt' cigars (Johnson *et al.*, 1998; Golub and Johnson, 1994).

The analysis of DUF/ADAM data on the cocaine epidemic suggests two things. First, the need to evaluate the effectiveness of policy interventions on a local basis. Second, the need to supplement quantitative survey data with ethnographic field research (cf. McKeganey, 1995).

It is clear from DUF/ADAM data that cocaine misuse became widely dispersed in most, although not all, of the metropolitan centres of the USA. Other forms of drug epidemic, however, have been more restricted. One recent development has been a sharp increase of methamphetamine use in the 1990s – with as many as 40 per cent of arrestees testing positive in San Diego – but this is entirely restricted to eight programme sites, all located on the Western seaboard and Southwestern States (NIJ, 1998). Elsewhere, positive methamphetamine tests are currently at or close to zero, and the DUF/ADAM programme offers an effective means to monitor the progress of this epidemic and offer early-warning signs of any eastward drift.

If the regional methamphetamine epidemic is recent, heroin misuse in the USA conforms to a pattern established by the heroin epidemic of the late 1960s and early 1970s. DUF/ADAM data throughout the 1980s and 1990s have consistently shown positive tests for heroin to be much lower and more localised than those for cocaine, hovering around 10 per cent in 8 cities, and reaching a high of 20 per cent only in Chicago and Manhattan, New York (NIJ, 1998; Riley, 1997). DUF/ADAM confirms that positive tests for heroin are much more likely to be found among older arrestees, although a few sites (New Orleans, Philadelphia and St Louis) are showing evidence of younger cohorts of heroin users, amidst fears that a new heroin epidemic could be under way (NIJ, 1998, p. 2; Inciardi and Harrison, 1998). Ethnographic fieldwork in St Louis and in New York's East Harlem offers some evidence of a shift from crack-cocaine to heroin among some users (Jacobs, 1999; Bourgois, 1995). The more consistent trend, however, is for an ageing cohort of opiate users, with an outreach study in New York, Chicago and San Diego, showing that one-third of a sample of current heroin users had first used heroin in a five-year period between 1968 and 1973: 'This is powerful testimony to the importance of avoiding heroin epidemics; a quarter-century after the last heroin epidemic, we are still dealing with its consequences' (Boyum and Rochelau, 1994, pp. 17–18).

Quite apart from any other considerations, the now well-established DUF/ADAM programme indicates the importance of estimating local and regional variations in patterns and levels of problem drug use for planning and delivering services. In the 'early warning' mechanism which DUF/ADAM offers, however imperfectly, of drug trends among a high-risk group of problem drug users unlikely to be currently in contact with services, it also offers a relatively cost-effective means of plotting regional variations in potential demand. Furthermore, it points to the comparative inadequacy of current drug monitoring provision in the UK.

Conclusion

It seems clear that some more proactive means of monitoring regional trends will need to be established if the periodic year-on-year evaluations of the UK government drug strategy are to have any real meaning. Given the emphasis in the strategy of targeting the most serious aspects of drug misuse, such as related criminality and anti-social nuisance, the DUF/ADAM programme would seem to offer a serviceable model. Moreover, if such a programme were calibrated in such a way as to offer direct comparability with the developing international ADAM programme, this might also offer an effective means of monitoring comparative European trends.

In summary, the evidence points clearly to the fact that drug epidemics do not move evenly through human populations. Rather, they tend to move in an uneven but consistent manner which inflicts the greatest damage on the poorest neighbourhoods. Drug problems therefore intersect with numerous other aspects of social exclusion and disadvantage – unemployment, housing decay, generally poorer levels of physical and mental health, etc. Where young people who grow up in these communities are concerned, as shown by a review of the research literature recently prepared for the UK government Social Exclusion Unit, problems of drug misuse are only one among many of the difficulties experienced by disaffected young people in poor neighbourhoods (Newburn, 1999). The wider context involves a variety of complex interlocking problems such as higher levels of truancy and exclusion from school, young people who hold few if any qualifications and work skills, together with the increased likelihood of having been 'looked after' in public care at some time (Newburn, 1999; Ward et al., 2003). Moreover, the review suggests that the most effective ways of responding to these difficulties are likely to be practical initiatives at a local level. The pressing need for drug services to be more effectively integrated within such local efforts becomes increasingly clear, and will no doubt be one of the major challenges of the UK government's newly fashioned drugs strategy.

References

Advisory Council on the Misuse of Drugs (1998). *Drug Misuse and the Environment*. London: HMSO.

Baumer, E., Lauritsen, J. L., Rosenfeld, R. and Wright, R. (1999). 'The Influence of Crack Cocaine on Robbery, Burglary and Homicide Rates: A Cross-City Longitudinal Analysis', *Journal of Research in Crime and Delinquency*, vol. 35, pp. 316–40.

Beck, J. and Rosenbaum, M. (1994). *Pursuit of Ecstasy: The MDMA Experience.* New York: State University of New York Press.

Bennett, T. (1998). *Drugs and Crime: The Results of Research on Drug Testing and Interviewing Arrestees.* Home Office Research Study 183. London: Home Office.

Bennett, T. (2000). *Drugs and Crime: The Results of the Second Developmental Stage of the NEW-ADAM Programme.* Home Office Research Study 205. London: Home Office.

Bottoms, A. E. and Wiles, P. (1986). 'Housing Tenure and Residential Crime Careers in Britain', in A. J. Reiss Jr. and M. Tonry, eds, *Communities and Crime, Crime and Justice: A Review of Research*, vol. 8. Chicago: University of Chicago Press, pp. 101–62.

Bottoms, A. E., Mawby, R. J. and Xanthos, P. (1989). 'A Tale of Two Estates', in D. Downes, ed., *Crime and the City: Essays in Memory of John Barron Mays.* London: Macmillan, pp. 36–97.

Bourgois, P. (1995). *In Search of Respect: Selling Crack in El Barrio.* Cambridge: Cambridge University Press.

Boyum, D. and Rocheleau, A. M. (1994). *Heroin Users in New York, Chicago, and San Diego.* Washington, DC: Office of National Drug Control Policy.

Burr, A. (1984). 'The Ideologies of Despair: A Symbolic Interpretation of Punks and Skinheads' Usage of Barbiturates', *Social Science and Medicine*, vol. 19, no. 9, pp. 929–38.

Burr, A. (1987). 'Chasing the Dragon: Heroin Misuse, Delinquency and Crime in the Context of South London Culture', *British Journal of Criminology*, vol. 27, pp. 333–57.

Chein, I., Gerard, D., Lee, R. and Rosenfeld, E. (1964). *The Road to H: Narcotics, Delinquency and Social Policy.* London: Tavistock.

Courtwright, D., Joseph, H. and Des Jarlais, D. (1989). *Addicts Who Survived: An Oral History of Narcotic Use in America, 1923–1965.* Knoxville: University of Tennessee Press.

Dai, B. (1937). *Opium Addiction in Chicago.* Chicago: University of Chicago Press.

De Alarcon, R. (1969). 'The Spread of Heroin Abuse in a Community', *Bulletin on Narcotics*, vol. 21, no. 3, pp. 17–22.

Faris, R. E. L. and Dunham, H. W. (1939). *Mental Disorder in Urban Areas.* Chicago: University of Chicago Press.

Fazey, C., Brown, P. J. B. and Batey, P. W. J. (1990). *A Socio-Demographic Analysis of Patients Attending in a Drug Dependency Clinic.* Working Paper 10, Urban Research and Policy Evaluation Regional Research Laboratory, University of Liverpool.

Feldman, H. W. (1968). 'Ideological Supports to Becoming and Remaining a Heroin Addict', *Journal of Health and Social Behaviour*, vol. 9, pp. 131–9.

Giggs, J., Bean, P., Whynes, D. and Wilkinson, C. (1989). 'Class A Drug Users: Prevalence Characteristics in Greater Nottingham', *British Journal of Addiction*, vol. 84, pp. 1473–80.

Gilman, M. (1988) 'DIY Diconal?', *Mersey Drugs Journal*, vol. 1, no. 5, p. 15.

Gilman, M. and Pearson, G. (1991). 'Lifestyles and Law Enforcement', in D. K. Whynes and P. T. Bean, eds, *Policing and Prescribing: The British System of Drug Control.* London: Macmillan, pp. 95–124.

Gilman, M., Traynor, P. and Pearson, G. (1990). 'The Limits of Intervention: Cyclizine Misuse', *Druglink*, vol. 5, no. 3, pp. 12–13.

Golub, A. and Johnson, B. D. (1994). 'A Recent Decline in Cocaine Use Among Youthful Arrestees in Manhattan (1987–1993)', *American Journal of Public Health*, vol. 84, no. 4, pp. 1250–4.

Golub, A. and Johnson, B. D. (1997). *Crack's Decline: Some Surprises Across U.S. Cities*. Washington, DC: National Institute of Justice.

Gore, S. (1999). 'Effective Monitoring of Young People's Use of Illegal Drugs: Meta-Analysis of UK Trends, and Recommendations', *British Journal of Criminology*, vol. 39, no. 4, pp. 575–84.

Hammersley, R., Ditton, J., Smith, I. and Short, E. (1999). 'Patterns of Ecstasy Use by Drug Users', *British Journal of Criminology*, vol. 39, no. 4, pp. 625–47.

Haw, S. (1985). *Drug Problems in Greater Glasgow*. London: SCODA.

Hough, M. and Mayhew, P. (1985). *Taking Account of Crime: Key Findings from the 1984 British Crime Survey*, Home Office Research Study no. 85. London: HMSO.

Hughes, P. H. (1977). *Behind the Wall of Respect: Community Experiments in Heroin Addiction Control*. Chicago: University of Chicago Press.

Hughes, P. H. and Crawford, G. A. (1972). 'A Contagious Disease Model for Researching and Intervening in Heroin Epidemics', *Archives of General Psychiatry*, vol. 27, pp. 189–205.

Hughes, P. H. and Rieche, O. (1995). 'Heroin Epidemics Revisited', *Epidemiological Reviews*, vol. 17, no. 1, pp. 66–73.

Hughes, P. H., Barker, N. W., Crawford, G. A. and Jaffe, J. H. (1972). 'The Natural History of a Heroin Epidemic', *American Journal of Public Health*, vol. 62, no. 7, pp. 995–1001.

Hunt, L. G. and Chambers, C. D. (1976). *The Heroin Epidemics: A Study of Heroin Use in the United States 1965–1975*. New York: Spectrum Books.

Inciardi, J. A. and Harrison, L. D., eds (1998). *Heroin in the Age of Crack Cocaine*. Thousand Oaks: Sage.

Jacobs, B. A. (1999). 'Crack to Heroin: Drug Markets in Transition?', *British Journal of Criminology*, vol. 39, no. 4, pp. 557–74.

Johnson, B. D., Goldstein, P. J., Preble, E., Schmeidler, J., Lipton, D. S., Spunt, B. and Miller, T. (1985). *Taking Care of Business: The Economics of Crime by Heroin Abusers*. Lexington: Lexington Books.

Johnson, B. D., Dunlap, E. and Sifaneck, S. J. (1998). 'The Blunted Generation: Changed Drug Use Patterns and Inner-City Isolation', American Society of Criminology Annual Meeting, Washington, DC, 11–14 November 1998.

Leitner, M., Shapland, J. and Wiles, P. (1993). *Drug Usage and Drugs Prevention: The Views and Habits of the General Public*. London: HMSO.

Lewis, R., Hartnoll, R., Bryer, S., Daviaud, E. and Mitcheson, M. (1985). 'Scoring Smack: The Illicit Heroin Market in London, 1980–1983', *British Journal of Addiction*, vol. 80, pp. 280–91.

Maher, L. (1997). *Sexed Work: Gender, Race and Resistance in a Brooklyn Drug Market*. Oxford: Oxford University Press.

McKeganey, N. (1995). 'Quantitative and Qualitative Research in the Addictions: An Unhelpful Divide', *Addiction*, vol. 90, no. 6, pp. 749–65.

McKeganey, N. and Barnard, M. (1992). *AIDS, Drugs and Sexual Risk: Lives in the Balance*. Buckingham: Open University Press.

Mirza, H. S., Pearson, G. and Phillips, S. (1991). *Drugs, People and Services in Lewisham: Final Report of the Drug Information Project*. London: Goldsmiths' College, University of London.

Munoz, L. and Davis, F. (1969). 'Heads and Freaks: Patterns and Meanings of Drug Use Among Hippies', *Journal of Health and Social Behaviours*, vol. 9, pp. 156–64.

National Institute of Justice (1988). *Drug Use Forecasting (DUF), Fourth Quarter 1988*. Washington, DC: National Institute of Justice.

National Institute of Justice (1997). *Drug Use Forecasting 1996: Annual Report on Adult and Juvenile Arrestees*. Washington, DC: National Institute of Justice.

National Institute of Justice (1998). *ADAM: 1997 Drug Use Forecasting. Annual Report on Adult and Juvenile Arrestees*. Washington, DC: National Institute of Justice.

Newburn, T. (1999). *Disaffected Young People in Poor Neighbourhoods. A Review of the Literature*. Unpublished report to the Social Exclusion Unit. London: Goldsmiths' College, University of London.

Nurco, D. N. (1972). 'An Ecological Analysis of Narcotic Addicts in Baltimore', *International Journal of the Addictions*, vol. 7, pp. 341–53.

Nurco, D. N., Shaffer, J. W. and Cisin, I. H. (1984). 'An Ecological Analysis of the Interrelationships Among Drug Abuse and Other Indices of Social Pathology', *International Journal of the Addictions*, vol. 19, pp. 441–51.

Parker, H., Aldridge, J. and Measham, F. (1998). *Illegal Leisure: The Normalization of Adolescent Recreational Drug Use*. London: Routledge.

Parker, H., Bakx, K. and Newcombe, R. (1988). *Living With Heroin: The Impact of a Drugs 'Epidemic' on an English Community*. Milton Keynes: Open University Press.

Parker, H., Bury, C. and Egginton, R. (1998). *New Heroin Outbreaks Among Young People in England and Wales*. Crime Detection and Prevention Series, Paper 92. London: Home Office.

Pearson, G. (1987a). *The New Heroin Users*. Oxford: Basil Blackwell.

Pearson, G. (1987b). 'Social Deprivation, Unemployment and Patterns of Heroin Use', in N. Dorn and N. South, eds, *A Land Fit for Heroin?* London: Macmillan, pp. 62–94.

Pearson, G. (1992). 'The Role of Culture in the Drug Question', in M. Lader, G. Edwards and D. C. Drummond, eds, *The Nature of Alcohol and Drug Related Problems*. Society for the Study of Addiction Monograph No. 3. Oxford: Oxford University Press, pp. 109–32.

Pearson, G. (1994). 'Youth, Crime, and Society', in M. Maguire, R. Morgan and R. Reiner, eds, *The Oxford Handbook of Criminology*. Oxford: Clarendon Press, pp. 1161–206.

Pearson, G. (1995). 'Drugs and Deprivation', in J. W. T. Dickerson and G. V. Stimson, eds, *Health in the Inner City: Drugs in the City*, supplement to *The Journal of the Royal Society of Health*, pp. 80–6.

Pearson, G. (2001). 'Normal Drug Use: Ethnographic Fieldwork Among an Adult Network of Recreational Drug Users in Inner London', *Substance Use and Misuse*, vol. 36, nos 1 and 2, pp. 167–200.

Pearson, G. and Gilman, M. (1994). 'Local and Regional Variations in Drug Misuse: The British Heroin Epidemic of the 1980s', in J. Strang and M. Gossop, eds, *Heroin Addiction and Drug Policy: The British System*. Oxford: Oxford University Press, pp. 102–20.

Pearson, G. and Hobbs, D. (2001). *Middle Market Drug Distribution*. Home Office Research Study 227. London: Home Office.

Pearson, G. and Patel, K. (1998). 'Drugs, Deprivation and Ethnicity: Outreach Among Asian Drug Users in a Northern English City', *Journal of Drug Issues*, vol. 28, no. 1, pp. 199–224.

Pearson, G., Ditton, J., Newcombe, R. and Gilman, M. (1991). 'Everything Starts with an "E": An Introduction to Ecstasy Use by Young People in Britain', *Druglink*, vol. 6, no. 6, pp. 10–11.

Pearson, G., Gilman, M. and McIver, S. (1985). *Young People and Heroin: An Examination of Heroin Use in the North of England*. London: Health Education Council.

Pearson, G., Mirza, H. S. and Phillips, S. (1993). 'Cocaine in Context: Findings from a South London Inner City Drug Survey', in P. Bean, ed., *Cocaine and Crack: Supply and Use*. London: Macmillan, pp. 99–129.

Peck, D. F. and Plant, M. A. (1986). 'Unemployment and Illegal Drug Use: Concordant Evidence from a Prospective Study and National Trends', *British Medical Journal*, vol. 293, pp. 929–32.

Power, A. (1997). *Estates on the Edge: The Social Consequences of Mass Housing in Northern Europe*. London: Macmillan.

Preble, E. and Casey, J. J. (1969). 'Taking Care of Business: The Heroin User's Life on the Street', *International Journal of the Addiction*, vol. 4, pp. 1–24.

President of the Council (1998). *Tackling Drugs to Build a Better Britain: The Government's 10-year Strategy for Tackling Drug Misuse*. Cm 3945. London: The Stationery Office.

Ramsay, M. and Percy, A. (1996). *Drug Misuse Declared: Results of the 1994 British Crime Survey*. Home Office Research Study no. 151. London: Home Office.

Ramsay, M. and Spiller, J. (1997). *Drug Misuse Declared in 1996: Latest Results from the British Crime Survey*. Home Office Research Study no. 172. London: Home Office.

Ramsay, M. and Partridge, S. (1999). *Drug Misuse Declared in 1998: Results from the British Crime Survey*. Home Office Research Study no. 197. London: Home Office.

Reuter, P., MacCoun, R. and Murphy, P. (1990). *Money from Crime: A Study of the Economics of Drug Dealing in Washington DC*. Santa Monica: RAND.

Reynolds, F. (1986). *The Problem Housing Estate*. Aldershot: Gower.

Riley, K. J. (1997). *Crack, Powder Cocaine, and Heroin: Drug Purchase and Use Patterns in Six U.S. Cities*. Washington, DC: National Institute of Justice and the Office of National Drug Control Policy.

Shaw, C. R. and McKay, H. D. (1942). *Juvenile Delinquency and Urban Areas*. Chicago: University of Chicago Press.

Stimson, G. V. and Oppenheimer, E. (1982). *Heroin Addiction*. London: Tavisock.

Taylor, A. (1993). *Women Drug Users: An Ethnography of a Female Injecting Community*. Oxford: Clarendon Press.

Taylor, A. (1998). 'Needlework: The Lifestyle of Female Drug Injectors', *Journal of Drug Issues*, vol. 28, no. 1, pp. 77–90.

Ward, J., Henderson, Z. and Pearson, G. (2003). *One Problem Among Many: Drug Use Among Care Leavers in Transition to Independent Living*. Home Office Research Study no. 260. London: Home Office.

Williams, T. (1989). *The Cocaine Kids*. New York: Addison-Wesley.

Williams, T. and Kornblum, W. (1985). *Growing Up Poor*. Lexington: Lexington Books.

Willis, P. (1978). *Profane Culture*. London: Routledge & Kegan Paul.

Wilson, A. R. (1999). *Urban Songlines: Subculture and Identity on the 1970s Northern Soul Scene*. Unpublished PhD Thesis. London: University of London.

Zinberg, N. E. (1984). *Drug, Set, and Setting: The Basis of Controlled Intoxicant Use*. New Haven: Yale University Press.

Chapter 10

The arrival of HIV

J. Roy Robertson

Since the Second World War, policy relating to management and treatment of drug abusers has been characterised by sudden upheavals followed by unplanned drifts in direction. Dramatic shifts in policy have resulted from political events, changing social structures and evolving medical philosophies rather than as a consequence of any advance in technology or understanding of the nature of the addictive disorder. Until its closure in 1997 probably the single most important determinant of interest in drug users has been the steady increase in numbers reported to the Home Office Addicts Index (Home Office 1997). Towards the end of 1985, however, events occurred which had probably the most dramatic impact on social policy in the latter half of the twentieth century – the identification of large numbers of known drug users as human immunodeficiency virus (HIV) antibody positive. This sudden discovery was brought about by the introduction of the laboratory test which could indicate the presence of antibodies in blood and, coming in the wake of the clinical epidemic of cases of acquired immune deficiency syndrome (AIDS) in homosexual men in the USA, its impact was tremendous.

Until this discovery the impact of AIDS or HIV among drug users had been minimal, although concerns were rapidly emerging in political and public health circles about the epidemic in the gay community (Garfield 1995). In the UK only seven cases of AIDS had been reported to the Public Health Laboratory Service (PHLS) by the end of 1985, four of these were also homosexual men. Each of the three injecting drug users who were not homosexual men travelled abroad and two certainly injected in Italy and the USA. In the fourth AIDS case whose only major risk factor was injecting drug use, there was no history of travel abroad. This case had a first positive HIV test in August 1985 and developed *Pneumocystis carinii* pneumonia (full-blown AIDS) in January 1986. All these cases were men.

By the end of 1985 a total of 55 reports of newly confirmed HIV infections in injecting drug users in England and Wales had been received. Two of these 55 had their positive specimens taken in November and December 1984. The remaining 53 were all tested in 1985. There is no information in surveillance data on earlier known positives and the positive tests discovered did not indicate for how long that individual might have been infected.

By the end of 1985, however, 356 positive test results attributable to intravenous drug use had been reported in Scotland (PHLS Colindale). It is reasonable to conclude from these findings that when the HIV test became generally available in 1985, HIV infection was already established in injecting drug users in Scotland, England and Wales. Transmission probably increased during 1982 and 1983 when a widespread epidemic of acute hepatitis B occurred amongst injecting drug users (Robertson 1985; McCormick *et al.* 1987). Retrospective testing in Scotland has shown that HIV was introduced in Edinburgh drug users in 1982 (Ronald *et al.* 1993; Burns *et al.* 1996). Rumours of the origins of the virus in the local drug-using population were various. The cities principally affected in Scotland were Edinburgh and Dundee. Glasgow, despite having a larger drug-using population, was apparently unaffected and any positive cases were attributed to drug users visiting from the east of the country to attend residential treatment services. Anxieties that the transmission from these individuals might cause a similar problem in the west led some physicians to recommend that they be treated outside the city. Possible sources of the Dundee problem seemed to point to Edinburgh. Whatever the introductory mechanism and further theories are discussed below, the conditions among injectors was right for rapid transmission. It is also important to note that not all drug users were infected by needle sharing. An unknown number were to reveal later that although they used drugs at the time they were never aware of sharing equipment under any circumstances likely to give rise to HIV transmission. A significant proportion of those infected are likely to have become infected by heterosexual intercourse.

Unlike the epidemic in the USA where cases of AIDS emerged rapidly subsequent to its discovery in 1981 the European and British experience was of the uncovering of a potential problem still some time in the future. This had important implications for the future development of research and clinical policy. Reading accounts of the early AIDS epidemic in the USA one is impressed by this difference (Jaffe *et al.* 1983; Shiltz 1987; Carrick 1989). Unlike the UK, several years elapsed before absolute confirmation was available of the cause of AIDS in the USA. In retrospect, therefore, it seems likely that HIV became endemic in the homosexual community in the USA in the mid- to late 1970s and that before long a substantial part of the intravenous drug-using population, at least in New York City, had become infected. This latter epidemic seems to have been greatly enhanced by the coincidental epidemic of intravenous cocaine-use (Schoenbaum *et al.* 1990). Some of this clearly extended to European centres and sporadic cases of AIDS occurred, therefore, among drug users in the UK prior to the availability of HIV antibody testing in 1985. In Scotland introduction may have been earlier and spread was certainly more rapid.

The impact of HIV antibody testing

A test to detect antibodies to HIV first became widely available throughout the developed countries in late 1985 and was initially applied to blood transfusion donations as this represented a major threat to an otherwise low-risk population. At the same time testing was carried out on samples from individuals thought to be at greater risk, including those using injecting drugs. In the UK testing of stored serum samples confirmed pilot studies on drug users which identified widespread infection in one or two centres (Peutherer *et al.* 1985; Robertson *et al.* 1986a; McClelland 1986). In a similar fashion testing in southern Europe identified a large problem among drug users, a clear indication of what would happen at some time in the future once the incubation period has elapsed. Patients and doctors alike were uncertain about the meaning of these results. Early disbelief was followed by acute anxiety and in some places panic about the potential epidemic and transmission possibilities. In 1996 there were very few symptomatic cases of AIDS or advanced HIV infection among drug users. Those who had a positive antibody test result were well, had few symptoms attributable to virus infection and little knowledge about the disease. Community anxiety about the disease and HIV transmission rapidly expanded to include medical facilities, local politicians, policy makers and the public. Everyone, including the media, was uncertain of the wider implications of HIV among drug users for the future.

Incubation time: the unique feature of HIV disease

Especially in 2004, it is difficult to understand the importance of our current knowledge of the long incubation period of AIDS. In addition in the early years of the AIDS epidemic no information was available to absolutely confirm that the disease was caused by a virus. In 1981 and 1982 it was suspected that this disease may have a prolonged incubation time, perhaps even 18 months, and it was a further two years before the disease was confirmed as being caused by a virus, named at the time HTLV-3 (due to its similarity to a group of viruses already known to be human pathogens). This was based on reported exposure times and the presence of many individuals who had clinical signs but remained otherwise well. Many medical people, therefore, suggested that not all those infected would become ill and that a chronic carrier state might exist without deteriorating health. As time went on it became more apparent that many of those infected would eventually become ill and that the incubation time might indeed be more prolonged than first imagined. The corollary, of course, was that infection might have been first introduced at an earlier stage and that research should look further back in time for the cause of the spread of the virus.

Even in 1985, when many Scottish drug users were found to be positive, the expectations were that 5 per cent of all those infected with HIV would eventually develop AIDS and that the remainder might remain in some chronic infected but moderately fit state. The subsequent three years were to rapidly eradicate this line of thought and increasingly depressing reports at subsequent World AIDS Conferences (Paris 1986; Washington 1987; Stockholm 1988) indicated the likelihood of the large majority of those with HIV antibodies to progress eventually to full AIDS. By the end of 1989, the understanding of the long incubation time was convincingly demonstrated (Moss *et al.* 1988) to be 10 years or longer. This has been further supported by a subsequent report of the progress of the San Francisco cohort which found the mean incubation period to be about 11 years. Nearly 20 per cent of this group were still well at the time of this report but continue to be under observation. Studies in haemophiliac cohorts have confirmed these findings although the passage of further time may even prolong this incubation time. Variations depending upon so-called 'cofactors' may lengthen or shorten incubation times in individuals and one important feature associated with length of time till the onset of symptomatic disease is the age at time of infection. Several studies may have indicated that those who become infected in older years may progress more quickly (Darby *et al.* 1989; Witcomb *et al.* 1990; Ronald *et al.* 1993).

This, therefore, makes clear many of the previous anomalies surrounding the natural cause of HIV infection. It also explains the slow emergence in some countries and indicates the difficulties in predicting the future. By the time cases of symptomatic AIDS come to the notice of clinicians the individual is likely to have been infected for up to 10 years and not only are the events of becoming infected obscured by time, but the possible transmission to subsequent drug using or sexual contacts may be enormous. Understanding this, therefore, is essential in order to contemplate the many routes the virus may have taken in the population both among drug users and sexual partners. It was not until 1996 that the first good news became available. In that year, at the XIth international AIDS conference in Vancouver, the scientific data confirming the efficacy of new antiviral chemotherapy was announced.

Edinburgh and Dundee

This, now familiar, HIV epidemic which occurred some time in the early 1980s remains the single most important source of knowledge of HIV infection in drug users in the UK. The introduction and implementation of the antibody test in Scotland rapidly indicated the presence of substantial numbers of infected drug users (Burns *et al.* 1996; Robertson 1986a). Case reports and positive tests throughout subsequent years accumulated over 1,000 individuals including sexual contacts and children (France *et al.* 1988; Mok *et al.* 1989). Individual cohorts were found to be extensively penetrated (Skidmore 1990) some 65 per cent or more being positive, comparable only with a few similarly damaged European and New York groups (Des Jarlais and Friedman 1987). A startlingly similar epidemic of HIV among the poor drug-using population of Dublin suggests similar problems to those in south-east Scotland and the pre-existing social and drug-using subculture describes identical conditions (O'Kelly 1998). Testing of old, stored, samples in Edinburgh, revealed infection present as far back as 1983 but no further, and the assumption is that HIV was introduced to this group at about that time. In order for spread to be so rapid certain conditions must have been present, including extensive needle and syringe sharing; accounts of drug use in these cities at that time is of a culture in which little care was taken to avoid the injections of blood from a previous user of the injecting equipment. Since that time, however, behaviour changes have been considerable, resulting in a progressive deterioration in numbers of individuals sharing equipment and a rapid increase in availability of needles and syringes from legal sources (Bury *et al.* 1996; Robertson 1989).

Although the extent of transmission is the distinguishing feature of the south-east Scotland epidemic, possibly more significant is the speed with which things happened. Within the space of 18 months or two years a substantial proportion of those injecting drugs had become infected, and after this transmissions slowed down dramatically. This may be due to several causes including the change in behaviour but at the present time few seropositive reports are due to needle and syringe sharing (Communicable Disease Unit, Scotland 1990) and the leading cause of infection has become heterosexual contact (Ronald *et al.* 1993).

At the present time, several years after the first introduction of the virus in both Edinburgh and Dundee, cases of full-blown AIDS are now emerging rapidly. In addition many individuals are developing symptoms both physical and psychological related to HIV infection and these issues are dominating the available services. The advance of treatment, particularly since 1996, has become the major issue for all individual health workers who have patients with HIV infection. The availability of this and other prophylactic therapies has significantly affected the counselling of patients considering testing for antibodies. It is no longer possible to say that there is no available treatment and that testing might reasonably be delayed until the onset of symptoms. Treatment with early antiviral chemotherapy has the additional advantage of having fewer side-effects. The headache, nausea and anaemia associated with larger doses of zidovudine in more advanced cases often reduced compliance or made it necessary to stop treatment. The domination of the drug-using population by AIDS has had a profound impact on the provision of services and also on the drug scene in general.

Anecdotal accounts of the introduction of the virus to the Edinburgh drug-using population

Although the detection of the mode of introduction of the HIV agent into any population has little practical value once it has happened, there are lessons which may prevent similar spread elsewhere. There is certainly an academic interest in tracing early cases as these may be of value in the virological techniques of identifying different strains of virus and mutations as infection is transmitted. There is also an epidemiological importance attached to any study of the rapid dissemination of the virus in any population.

Several accounts have emerged of drug users travelling and sharing equipment with contacts in southern European centres. The most clearly defined example illustrates an individual known to be an early positive in Edinburgh who had used extensively in a Spanish centre (Bisset *et al.* 1989). Other studies include contacts with drug-using homosexual American servicemen in England and linkage by way of a drug-injecting man known to have haemophilia. Accounts of drug-using Americans in Scotland have been unsubstantiated but extensive links with Amsterdam and occasionally Dublin raise other possibilities. An itinerant Scot who spent several years in California, including a long prison sentence, before returning to injecting drug use in Edinburgh may be the introductory contact.

Other accounts of the drug subculture at the time when HIV is thought to have been introduced are various but one interesting story told by a long-standing drug-dependent patient gives an interesting version of events from the perspective of an individual heavily involved with using drugs at the same time as supplying them to others (the *J.F.K.* referred to is the US navy ship visiting at the time).

> I don't remember the exact year but it would be late '70s when the *J.F.K.* anchored in the Forth for a few weeks, with over a thousand men on board. At that time, I was handling sales at this side of Edinburgh for the 'Pharmacy Busters'. The more I sold the more I could use myself. I made my way to the docks as soon as the crew landed. It was only minutes before I was leaving with a carload of Americans, all desperate for a hit of heroin, morphine, cocaine or anything else for that matter. I take five of them back to my house to 'taste the wares'. There are two 'house' 'sets of works' and five spikes, which have been in use for a couple of months. They use them because they don't have their own. The 'sets' then go on to be used for several more months by God knows everyone. (I had my own.) I elected two guys to come and score for the rest of the users. They were buying up to 12 grams of 'H' or morphine and 12 grams of cocaine and some other drugs, enough for about 2,500 hits by my reckoning, every 2–3 days. I was told there are a few 'sets' on

board in covert places where the users could have a hit, then clean and replace the 'sets' for the next person.

There were hundreds of crewmen who went with the mostly 'H'-addicted prostitutes. They would ask the girls to get them bags of 'H' and share it with them, as well as sharing the girls' 'sets'. The men went back aboard and obviously had to use the 'covert' works for their share of the 'H' etc., previously scored by the 'selected two'. The girls in turn went home to share their 'sets' with their partners and friends.

The *J.F.K.* put in at Portsmouth around a year later and the guys were back on my doorstep again. 'Hi man, what you got for us?' They did not have their own 'sets' and told me that the 'covert' sets were brutally blunt and stiff and were in fact the same ones that had been there since they boarded!

Many drug users who were actively injecting during the early 1980s (when HIV is known to have been introduced into this group) remain convinced that the mode of introduction was through sexual contacts with prostitutes working in the dock area of Edinburgh. Many of these young women were drug users and this is considered by some to be the most likely mode of introduction to the drug-using subculture of Edinburgh. Clearly many prostitutes will have contacts with itinerants and overseas visitors and this certainly could be one explanation for the presence of HIV in Edinburgh. Links with Dundee were well established, drug users visiting Dundee on a regular basis to obtain quantities of heroin, some injecting in Edinburgh, and some taking drugs home to be redistributed in that city. Of some interest and importance is the position of buprenorphine (Temgesic) as a drug of injection as this emerged rapidly as a popular drug of abuse during 1984 and 1985 when it became available in tablet form and was prescribed by general practitioners. Prior to that this drug had been used extensively in hospital practice as a drug of injection for pain killing, usually post-operatively. After introduction as a tablet, it rapidly became widely abused (Robertson and Bucknall 1986b) and since then has enjoyed a position of some popularity amongst drug users throughout the UK. The significance of this drug is its comparatively short-term action when injected intravenously and the consequent excessive use in the course of a day. Thus drug users might inject up to ten times per day a drug which has a short action rather than the two or three injections usually used with heroin. The coincidence of an epidemic of Temgesic abuse round about the time of introduction of HIV is similar to the cocaine problems reported in the United States, especially New York, which were thought to account for the rapid spread of HIV in that city (Schoenbaum *et al.* 1990).

Whatever the introductory event, the graphic descriptions of injecting techniques in Edinburgh at that time go a long way to explaining why transmission occurred so completely and rapidly. The abrupt closure of the most important distributor of new sterile injecting equipment in September 1982 led almost immediately to an extensive needle- and syringe-sharing group (Henderson 1985: unpublished personal account of the Bread Street Shop 1980–82). A well-documented epidemic of hepatitis B followed the closure of this supply of injecting equipment. Repeated accounts of groups using large 10 or 20 ml syringes are recorded (Robertson and Bucknall 1986a). At these times a strong solution of heroin was mixed and drawn into a syringe, serial individuals would stick the needle into a vein, draw back blood to confirm that it was in the vein, inject 2–5 ml of solution and withdraw the needle. The syringe and needle, plus increasing mixtures of blood, would then be passed on to the next user. Many individuals clearly recall the presence of 20 or 30 individuals at such sessions. It is easy to imagine transmission occurring epidemically under these conditions. Evidence suggests that these extreme patterns of drug use largely disappeared around 1985. The descriptions of so-called shooting galleries from New York was appropriate for the conditions in Edinburgh and Dundee in late 1980 and throughout 1981. Sharing equipment among drug users is always common and persists to the present time with the consequent spread of blood-borne viruses. Even in 1998 there are reports of hepatitis C virus spread by this route. Spread of hepatitis B and hepatitis C are now known to be prevalent in most drug-using groups studied (the latter at a higher rate than the former) and the presumption is that the majority of this infection is due to shared injecting paraphernalia. HIV infection has penetrated drug-using communities differently or not at all. The conclusion that it is harder to transmit this virus than the hepatitis viruses is based on cumulative evidence over many years and reports of preferential infection by hepatitis. Sharing conditions adequate for the passage of hepatitis may not be so for the transmission of HIV. The behaviour necessary for transmission in epidemic form may not be present in many drug-using centres. Certainly the extreme levels of exchange of blood from person to person witnessed in the epidemic years in Edinburgh have not often been described. This arose from the rapidity of and emerging epidemic of drug use in a young population with little or no knowledge combined with a ruthless suppression of drug-using activities by the law-enforcement authorities and a lack of concern by the health services.

Molecular epidemiolgy

Using techniques which sequence the genetic codes of the virus, or parts of the virus, similarities and differences can be shown between virus cultures from blood taken from different individuals. In those infected from a common origin, sequences will be similar and this similarity will increase if the infection occurred at a similar time. Types or strains of HIV 1 have been identified in various countries and have shown characteristics which make them divisible into various groups. These groups or subtypes can identify a sample as originating from Africa or North America. Further subdivisions can identify connections between samples giving rise to conclusions about the historical spread of the virus and geographical connections.

Such techniques have shown close links between drug users from Edinburgh with those from Dundee, confirming the impression that these two cities experienced introduction of HIV at the same time. Further similarities have been shown with samples from infected drug users in Dublin, a pattern suggesting a recent common origin (Leigh Brown *et al.* 1997). In nearly 200 patients from Edinburgh and Dundee and 200 from Dublin there was little overlap with samples taken from gay men. Although there were a few gay men who had drug-using-type sequences (presumably because they acquired the infection from injecting drugs), the pattern suggested a separate origin, as did the sequencing of a small number of injecting drug users from Belfast (where the number of drug users is small). In Glasgow and Newcastle samples showed similar patterns to Edinburgh and Dundee but all were markedly different from the pattern found in London, where gay men and drug users had differences suggesting a separate origin. European comparisons showed Amsterdam to have similar types of virus to those in Edinburgh and Dundee. France and Sweden had 50 per cent similar to Edinburgh and Dundee. Sequencing from Spain, Portugal and Italy were all quite different, suggesting a separate source. Both these separate northern and southern European epidemics are probably closer to North America than African types (none are similar to African types).

Thailand studies showed, interestingly, that the virus changed over the course of the epidemic. Early samples from Bangkok were similar to the North American subtype B. The E subtype spread rapidly among heterosexuals and established the epidemic in Chiang Mai which then spread to Bangkok, leading to mixed B and E in Bangkok (Kalish *et al.* 1995).

Drug services: changing priorities

The statements of the 1986 Scottish Committee and the subsequent Advisory Council on the Misuse of Drugs (ACMD) Reports (McClelland 1986; ACMD 1988, 1989) to the effect that the prevention of AIDS was more important than the prevention of drug injecting to a certain extent set the scene for subsequent changes in available services. Whether or not this re-medicalisation of drug misuse stands the test of time remains to be seen but at a stroke the attitude of the establishment had changed. Over the next few years a dramatic growth of services targeted at implementing the new philosophy emerged. Needle exchange from clinics, general practice services, mobile units and pharmacies became regular features and prescribing substitute drugs for those dependent was transformed from a shady pastime advocated by a few to a well-supported clinical priority led by physicians and psychiatrists. Educational campaigns both national and local prioritised drug users and latterly heterosexual partners as targets for safe drug use and safe-sex campaigns. Widespread media coverage made AIDS a household issue and its association with intravenous drug use unquestioned. Political endorsement of needle and syringe exchange followed somewhat reluctantly in both England and Scotland with the rising panic about the potential for drug users to spread HIV into the wider heterosexual community. The heat generated in government and among academics is well described in two separated historical accounts of the HIV epidemic (Berridge 1998; Garfield 1995). The importance of HIV in forming subsequent national and international drug policy cannot be overestimated and in the era of awareness of hepatitis C is forgotten at our peril (see Chapter 17, this volume).

The rapid spread of HIV in south-east Scotland was initially thought to presage similar discoveries in other UK cities, and several attempts have been made to identify the scale of the problem in other regions. Surprisingly, no such problem has yet been found in any other centre including cities with a substantially larger drug misuse problem than either Edinburgh or Dundee. These include Glasgow, Liverpool and London where studies have included a low seroprevalence for HIV antibodies among drug users (PHLS 1990; Communicable Disease Service Unit, Scotland 1990). Additional studies of pregnant women and new-born children may supply more information shortly and Medical Research Council studies of anonymous samples from various centres are currently under way. Looking further afield, however, it becomes apparent that many other centres with large long-established drug-using subcultures have low or slowly rising rates of HIV infection. These include Amsterdam, California and London (Buning 1986; Watters 1988). Moreover, the global AIDS epidemic is dominated in pure numerical terms by heterosexual transmission, this population obviously being the biggest risk group of all. Sexual spread among men and women seems to emerge slowly after the introduction of the infection to a population reaching large numbers after several years (Ancelle 1990; Chin 1990). Implementation of what came to be known as harm-minimisation policies in the late 1980s may indeed have diverted a larger epidemic of HIV among UK drug injectors and their sexual partners (Stimson 1996; see also Chapter 16, this volume). Recent revelations about hepatitis C transmission may, however, require further scrutiny of safe practices (Wodak 1998).

Managing drug users post-AIDS

In the new climate of post-AIDS awareness by both drug workers and drug users things may or may not have changed. Drug injecting clearly continues and abusers reported to the National Surveillance System increase year by year (Home Office 1997). Neither has needle sharing vanished despite the new availability of equipment (Donoghoe *et al.* 1989). The initial emergence of new services in the late 1980s has clearly been a positive spin-off from knowledge of AIDS by the establishment, but in areas outside those known to have large numbers of infected individuals this may not be sustained and in those areas with a lot of infected individuals new services tend understandably to be dominated by clinical AIDS issues. At the beginning of this chapter the characteristics of changes in drug policy were discussed and the tendency for a shift in policy and service provision to be followed by a gradual drift in policy and slackening in enthusiasm for support. The gradual withdrawal of funds often is the key determinant of the failure of projects to work or policies to be effective. The awareness of AIDS has been associated with rapid development of new services but the most important issue for the next decade is to sustain these services. For this reason it is crucial that service provisions are not fragmented and that overlap between agencies is minimal. Drug users with or without HIV infection require therapies of various types and this is merely complicated by the presence of HIV. HIV and AIDS are here to stay and have opened up new responsibilities for drug workers and medical staff. Because of the presence of HIV infection drug misuse has undoubtedly been taken more seriously than before. Perhaps this is because those infected by drug taking represent a bridge into the general population by way of heterosexual spread (Wyld *et al.* 1997a). It will certainly take many years or even decades to understand the full implications of HIV infection among drug users (Friedland and Klein 1987). Those workers familiar with the emerging problems of those infected in Scotland have no doubts about the seriousness of these possibilities and already understand the devastating effect HIV and AIDS have on individuals and families.

Non-AIDS HIV illness

Studies in New York City (Stoneburner *et al.* 1988) have illustrated the non-opportunistic infections associated with HIV infections. It seems that prior to the onset of full-blown AIDS those individuals are susceptible to a range of infectious diseases and other conditions not necessarily related to advanced immune dysfunction. Bacterial pneumonia, meningitis, tuberculosis, and other infections may cause illness or sudden death. In addition the frequency of lethal overdose seems greater in those infected. Clearly this latter cause of death is possibly deliberate (suicide) but an increased susceptibility to overdose may arise from reduced respiratory function. Mortality and ongoing illness from many causes will obviously increase in the drug-using population infected with HIV (Shishodia *et al.* 1998).

The new European definition of AIDS (Ancelle-Park 1993) takes in some of these HIV-related illnesses and will increase the numbers included as advanced disease. This has some importance for epidemiologists and in natural history studies.

Hepatitis

The rapid global problems associated with HIV infection in drug users has to some extent overshadowed the epidemics of hepatitis B and hepatitis C. Hepatitis C infection is universally more prevalent among injecting drug users than hepatitis B which is more common than HIV infection. The so-called flaviviruses seem to be more easily transmitted by even minor breeches of infection control guidelines than HIV. In countries like the UK and Australia where injecting equipment is readily available, hepatitis C in particular continues to spread rapidly although in most centres HIV is uncommon (Wodak 1998). Co-infection with hepatitis B and C and HIV carries a worse prognosis than any one virus on its own. The high prevalence of hepatitis C gives rise to anxieties about vertical transmission from mother to baby either in utero, at birth or by breast feeding. In PCR-negative mothers these risks appear to be low (Johnstone 1998).

Developing new services to manage HIV infection in drug users

Rapidly changing events have altered the philosophical basis of delivering services to drug users and have also altered those involved in these organisations. A return to a medical model of care has required that more physicians are now influential in providing hospital care especially for those with HIV infection. General practitioners and psychiatrists are similarly increasingly in contact with drug users and encouraged to provide appropriate levels of intervention. As well as these agencies there has been extensive growth in the non-statutory sector and a new imperative for liaison between agencies.

These changes in perspective caused by HIV and the involvement of a wider range of medical professionals has had different effects in different regions of the UK. A return to the abstinence model of therapy has rather unfortunately dominated much of the recent discussion and in many major drug-using centres services are available on this basis only. Regrettably the wide range of necessary services advocated by many to supply the needs of continuing drug users and those who are not able to abstain are not available in many areas despite the presence of HIV infection and AIDS. The next few years are likely to see much jostling for position among agencies trying to secure continuing funding and all those interested need to ensure the development of all agencies. The non-statutory sector is particularly vulnerable and suffers most from the pressures and stresses of short-term funding.

All agencies now becoming familiar with HIV-infected and AIDS-suffering drug users are aware of the incredible range of problems which become regular features. Moreover, the prospect of large numbers of symptomatic drug users living with AIDS for many years is, to say the least, intimidating for those planning such services.

Since 1996 death rates have fallen sharply across Europe. According to data in the *Lancet* (1998, vol. 352: 1725–30) between 1995 and 1998 rates dropped from 23 to 4 deaths per 100 person-years of follow-up, a fall of more than 80 per cent. The investigators attribute these dramatic results to new combinations of treatment, but point out that they apply to only 2 per cent of the world's HIV sufferers. The rest live and die outside Europe and North America. Preventing infection has always been acclaimed as the best treatment and for injecting drug users there is much to suggest that a combination of education treatment and provision of conditions which reduce the likelihood of needle, syringe and other injecting paraphernalia has prevented the predicted caseload (Stimson 1996).

Acknowledgements

I would like to acknowledge help given by Dr Noel Gill (PHLS) and Professor David Goldberg (SCIEH) in preparation of the surveillance data in this chapter. The paragraphs on molecular epidemiology are as a result of help from Andrew Leigh Brown at Edinburgh University.

References

ACMD (Advisory Council on the Misuse of Drugs) (1988). *AIDS and drug misuse*, Part 1. HMSO, London.

ACMD. (1989). *AIDS and drug misuse*, Part 2. Report by the Advisory Council on the Misuse of Drugs. HMSO, London.

Ancelle, J. (1990). All Party Parliamentary Committee Occasional Paper No. 1. London.

Ancelle-Park, R. (1993). Expanded European AIDS case definition (letter). *Lancet*, 341: 1440–1.

Angarano, G., Pastore, G., Monno, L., Santantonio, T., Luchena, N. and Schiraldi, O. (1985). Rapid spread of HTLVIII infection among drug addicts in Italy. *Lancet*, ii: 1302.

Berridge, V. (1998) 1986. The drugs issue. AIDS rises up the policy agenda. In V. Berridge, ed., *AIDS in the UK. The making of policy, 1981–1994*. Oxford University Press, Oxford, 81–99.

Bisset, C., Jones, G., Davidson, J., Cummins, B., Burns, S., Inglis, J. M. and Brettle, R. P. (1989). Mobility of injection drug users and transmission of HIV. *Lancet*, ii: 44.

Brettle, R. P., Bisset, K., Burns, S., Davidson, J., Davidson, S. J. and Gray, J. M. N. (1987). Human immunodeficiency virus and drug misuse: the Edinburgh experience. *British Medical Journal*, 295: 421–4.

Buning, E. (1990). The role of harm reduction programmes in curbing the spread of HIV by drug injections. In G. Stimson and J. Strang, eds, *AIDS and drug misuse*, Routledge, London, 153–61.

Burns, S. M., Brettle, R. P., Gore, S. M., Peutherer, J. P. and Robertson, J. R. (1996). The epidemiology of HIV infection in Edinburgh related to the injecting of drugs: an historical perspective and new insight regarding the past incidence of HIV infection derived from retrospective HIV antibody testing of stored samples of serum. *Journal of Infection*, 32: 53–62.

Bury, J. K., Ross, A., van Teijlingen, F., Porter, A. M. and Bath, G. (1996). Lothian general practitioners, HIV infection and drug misuse: epidemiology, experience and confidence 1988–1993. *Health Bulletin*, 54, 3: 258–69.

Carrick, P. (1989). AIDS: ethical, legal and public policy implications. In E. T. Juengst and B. A. Koening, eds, *The meaning of AIDS*, Praeger, New York, 163–73.

Chin, I. (1990). All Party Committee on AIDS. Occasional Paper I. House of Commons. Communicable Disease Surveillance Unit (Scotland) (1990). Monthly report, September. Ruchill, Glasgow.

Darby, S. C., Rizza, C. R., Doll, R., Spooner, R. J. D., Stratton, I. M. and Thakrar, B. (1989). Incidence of AIDS and excess mortality associated with HIV in haemophiliacs in the United Kindom: report on behalf of the directors of haemophilia centres in the United Kingdom. *British Medical Journal*, 298: 1064–8.

Des Jarlais, D. C. and Friedman, S. R. (1987). Editorial review: HIV infection among intravenous drug users: epidemiology and risk reduction. *AIDS*, 1: 67–76.

Donoghoe, M. C., Stimson, G. V., Dolan, K. and Alldritt, L. (1989). Changes in HIV risk behaviour in clients of syringe-exchange schemes in England and Scotland. *AIDS*, 3(5): 267–72.

France, A. J., Skidmore, C. A., Robertson, J. R., Brettle, R. P., Roberts, J. J. K., Burns, S. M., *et al.* (1988). Heterosexual spread of HIV in Edinburgh. *British Medical Journal*, 296: 526–9.

Friedland, G. H. and Klein, R. (1987). Transmission of the human immunodeficiency virus. *New England Journal of Medicine*, 317: 1125–35.

Garfield, S. (1995) *The end of innocence. Britain in the time of AIDS*, Faber & Faber, London.

Home Office. (1997). Statistics of the misuse of drugs: addicts notified to the Home Office, UK, 1996. HMSO, London.

Jaffe, H. W., Bregman, D. J. and Selik, R. M. (1983). Acquired immune deficiency syndrome in the United States: the first 1,000 cases. *Journal of Infectious Diseases*, 148: 339–45.

Johnstone, F. D. (1998). Pregnant drug users. In J. R. Robertson, ed., *Management of drug users in the community*, Arnold. London.

Kalish, M. L., Baldwin, A., Raktham, S., Wasi, C., Luo, C. C., Schochetman, G., Mastro, T. D., Young, N., Vanichsensi, S., Rubsamen-Waigmann, H. *et al.* (1995). The evolving molecular epidemiology of HIV-1 envelope subtypes injecting drug users in Bangkok, Thailand: implications for HIV vaccine trials. *AIDS* 9, 8: 851–7.

Lazzarin, A., Galli, M., Geroldi, D., Zanetti, A., Crocchiolo, P. and Aiuti, F. (1985). Epidemic of LAV/HTLVIII infection in drug addicts in Milan: serological survey and clinical follow-up. *Infection*, 13, 5: 216–18.

Leigh Brown, A. J., Lobidel, D., Wade, C. M., Rebus, S., Phillips, A. N., Brettle, R. P., France, A. J., Leen, C. S., McMenamin, J., McMillan, A., Maw, R. D., Mulcahy, F., Robertson, J. R., Sankar, K. N., Scott, G., Wyld, R. and Peutherer, J. F. (1997). The molecular epidemiology of human immunodeficiiency virus type 1 in six cities in Britain and Ireland. *Virology*, 235: 166–77.

McClelland, D. B. L. (1986). *HIV infection in Scotland*. Report of the Scottish Committee on HIV Infection and Intravenous Drug Use. SHHD, Edinburgh.

McCormick, A., Tillet, H., Bannister, B. and Emslie, J. (1987). Surveillance of AIDS in the United Kingdom. *British Medical Journal*, 295: 1466–9.

Mok, Y. J. O., Hague, R. A., Yap, P. L., Hargreaves, F. D., Inglis, J. M. and Whitelaw, J. M. (1989). Vertical transmission of HIV: a prospective study. *Archives of Disease in Childhood*, 64: 1140–5.

Morgan Thomas, R. (1990). AIDS risks, alcohol, drugs and the sex industry: a Scottish study. In M. Plant, ed., *AIDS, drugs and prostitution*, Routledge, London, 88–108.

Moss, A. R., Bacchetti, P., Osmond, D., Krampf, W., Chaisson, R. E. and Sittes, D. (1988). Seropositivity for HIV and the development of AIDS or AIDS related condition: three year follow up of the San Francisco General Hospital cohort. *British Medical Journal*, 296: 745–50.

O'Kelly, F. D. (1998). HIV/AIDS care and management. In J. R. Robertson, ed., *Management of drug users in the community*, Arnold, London, 172–92.

Peutherer, J. F., Edmond, E., Simmonds, P., Dickson, J. D. and Bath, G. (1985). HTLV-III antibody in Edinburgh drug addicts. *Lancet*, ii: 1129–30.

PHLS (1990). AIDS Centre. Quarterly unpublished reports. No. 8, September, Colindale, London.

Robertson, J. R. (1985). Drug users in general practice. *British Medical Journal*, 290: 34–5.

Robertson, J. R. and Bucknall, A. B. V. (1986a). *Heroin users in a Scottish city*. SHHD, Edinburgh.

Robertson, J. R. and Buchnall, A. B. V. (1986b). Buprenorphine – dangerous drug or overlooked therapy (letter). *British Medical Journal*, 292: 1465.

Robertson, J. R. and Skidmore, C. A. (1989). *AIDS in the family*. Report to SHHD, Edinburgh.

Robertson, J. R., Bucknall, A. B. V., Welsby, P. D., Roberts, J. J. K., Inglis, J. M. and Brettle, R. P. (1986a). Epidemic of AIDS related virus (HTLV-III/LAV infection among intravenous drug abusers). *British Medical Journal*, 292: 527–9.

Ronald, P. J. M., Robertson, J. R. and Elton, R. A. (1994). Continued drug use and other cofactors for progression to AIDS among injecting drug users. *AIDS*, 8: 339–43.

Ronald, P. J. M., Robertson, J. R., Wyld, R. and Weightman, R. (1993). Heterosexual transmission of HIV in injecting drug users. *British Medical Journal*, 307: 1184–5.

Rutherford, G. W., Lifson, A. R., Hessol, N. A., Darrow, W. W., O'Malley, P. M., Buckbinder, S. P. *et al.* (1990). Course of HIV-1 infection in a cohort of homosexual and bisexual men: an 11 year follow up study. *British Medical Journal*, 301: 1183–8.

Schoenbaum, E. E., Hartel, D., Selwyn, P. A., Klein, R. S., Davenny, K., Rogers, M., Feiner, C. and Friedland, G. (1990). Risk factors for human immunodeficiency virus infection in intravenous drug users. *New England Journal of Medicine*, 322: 632–3.

Shiltz, R. (1987). *And the band played on*. Penguin. London.

Shishodia, P., Robertson, J. R. and Milne, A. (1998). Causes and frequency of deaths in injecting drug users between 1981 and 1997 in Edinburgh. *Scottish Office Health Bulletin* 56, 2: 553–6.

Skidmore, C. A., Robertson, J. R. and Elton, R. A. (1990). After the epidemic: follow up study of HIV seroprevalence and changing patterns of drug use. *British Medical Journal*, 300: 219–23.

Stimson, G. V. (1996). Has the United Kingdom averted an epidemic of HIV-1 infection amongst drug injectors? Editorial. *Addiction*, 91, 8: 1085–8.

Stimson, G. V., Alldrit, L. and Dolan, K. (1988). Syringe exchange schemes for drug users in England and Scotland. *British Medical Journal*, 296: 1717–19.

Stimson, G. V., Hunter, G. M., Donoghoe, M. C., Rhodes, T., Parry, J. V. and Chalmers, C. P. (1996). HIV-1 prevalence in community-wide samples of injecting drug users in London, 1990–1993. *AIDS*, 10, 6: 657–66.

Stoneburner, R. L., Des Jarlais, D. C., Benezra, D., Gorelkin, L., Southern, J. L., Friedman, S. R. *et al.* (1988). A larger spectrum of severe HIV-1 related disease in intravenous drug users in New York City. *Science*, 242: 916–19.

Watters, J. K., Case, P., Huang, Cheng, Y. T., Lorvick, J. and Carlson, J. (1988). *HIV seropositivity and behavioural changes in intravenous drug users.* Poster at IVth International Conference on AIDS, June 1988, Stockholm.

Witcomb, J. C., Skidmore, C. A., Roberts, J. J. K. and Elton, R. A. (1990). Progression to AIDS in intravenous drug users, cofactors and survival. IVth International AIDS Conference, San Francisco.

Wodak, A. (1998). Medical complications of drug taking. In J. R. Robertson, ed., *Management of drug users in the community.* Arnold. London.

Wyld, R., Robertson, J. R. and Gillon, J. (1997a). Spread of HIV infection from non-drug user to non-drug user. *British Journal of General Practice*, 47: 595.

Wyld, R., Robertson, J. R., Brettle, R. P., Mellor, J., Prescott, L. and Simmonds, P. (1997b). Absence of HCV transmission but frequent transmission of HIV-1 from sexual contact with doubly infected individuals. *Journal of Infection*, 35: 163–6.

Chapter 11

The great Mersey experiment
The birth of harm reduction

Peter McDermott

Introduction: notes on method

The narrative that follows is, in part at least, a personal account of how an unlikely group of people sought to challenge the current assumptions and the dominant view of British drug policy at that time, with the aim of replacing it with their own, and in doing so, achieved a level of success that was way beyond any they could have ever imagined possible.

Towards the end of the 1980s, a number of drugs agencies on Merseyside adopted a new model of thinking about and responding to drugs problems. With backing from the local police and the regional health authority, this policy of 'harm reduction' was, in many ways, a complete U-turn from the trajectory British drug policy and treatment philosophy had been taking for the previous twenty years, and for some of the architects of the policy, was a conscious and explicit attempt to roll back the current paradigm for dealing with drug problems to the classic principles that underpinned the original British System as outlined by the Rolleston and Brain committees.

This chapter will look at the political and social context within which the Merseyside experiment took place, examine some of the strengths and weaknesses of the theory and practice that underpinned that model, and attempt to see if any lessons can be drawn from the experience.

The background to the experiment in Merseyside

By the late 1970s, there was widespread disillusionment with the old British System, and a change of direction was inevitable. The system had been subjected to an extremely effective attack by regressive forces who viewed opioid agonist maintenance as perpetuating dependence for much longer periods than was really necessary.

This faction argued that the majority of people who were seen by services were actually poly-drug abusers rather than the pure opiate addicts of the Rolleston era, and that their dependence was artificially extended by treatment. As opiate addiction wasn't actually life threatening, they argued, we really weren't doing our patients any favours by maintaining them indefinitely. Quite the contrary, we were actually doing them a disservice.

The old British System, their argument went, was grounded in a medical model of addiction that just wasn't supported by the available evidence. The real problems that these people faced tended to be a series of social problems as opposed to medical. Rather than having a consultant psychiatrist dominate the care of such people, it actually made far more sense to create multidisciplinary teams, in which the doctor was just one member of a team that included social workers, probation officers, welfare rights and housing workers – in short, a fully social approach to a social problem.

This model rapidly gained support, particularly when the thinking behind it informed the ACMD's report on Treatment and Rehabilitation in the early 1980s (ACMD, 1982). This document was to virtually abolish the practice of maintenance in the UK. Certainly maintenance on heroin and methadone ampoules became almost impossible to obtain for a new patient or a patient returning to treatment if they lived anywhere apart from a handful of treatment backwaters.

Merseyside was one such backwater.

A personal perspective

As a patient at most of these clinics during this period, my assessment and evaluation of them was far from being a disinterested one. Along with the other patients, I grumbled about the irrationality and arbitrary nature of service provision, and what I then regarded as the indefensible strategy to provide methadone maintenance rather than diamorphine. The only possible reason for adopting such an approach, as far as my cohort and I could see, was a moral one. Nevertheless, I was fairly content and happy with the treatment I received. After a few years, I began to stop bothering using non-prescribed drugs, and enrolled on a degree course.

Throughout this period, I was always conscious of a dark cloud looming on the horizon. Thirty miles down the road was Manchester, the nearest major city to Liverpool, and the birthplace of the new 'Community Drug Team' model of drug treatment provision. There, both new patients and old patients who had dropped out of treatment for whatever reason, found themselves subjected to the new regime. Where we considered ourselves fortunate to get our medication and minimal supervision, over in Manchester, you'd be unlikely to get any medication, but instead would receive plenty of group therapy. If you were lucky enough to persuade somebody to prescribe a methadone detoxification programme, it would usually last only a few weeks or a couple of months.

Among addict circles, it was felt that such services were a complete waste of time. These brief detoxification programmes were unlikely to succeed, as they just didn't give you enough time, and so people would stay in treatment until the dose dropped below the comfort level, and then they'd go – only to come back again the next time they were arrested or hit some other crisis. And if the chemotherapy was considered useless, the psychotherapy was regarded as risible. Nobody I ever talked to was ever able to see the purpose of the variants of humanistic psychotherapy that were offered up in place of medication, other than as some curious job creation scheme aimed at finding a role for the less talented members of the middle classes.

Like many other addicts on Merseyside, I regarded this situation as irrational, unfair and extremely threatening. I'd managed to secure some small degree of stability due to the maintenance regime that I was treated under. By the mid-1980s, I was sufficiently stable to have stopped using illicit drugs completely, and was studying for my master's degree. It seemed so unreasonable that if I'd lived just thirty miles down the road, in Manchester, if I wasn't able to manage to successfully detoxify and stay clean, I would have been condemned to a life of chaotic instability and continuous arrests. In an attempt to find some way to fight back against this threat, I decided to study drug policy. I might still be an unemployable drug addict after I graduated, but at least I'd have done as much as I possibly could have done to challenge this new paradigm and the threat that it posed to my sense of stability and wellbeing.

HIV, AIDS and the rebirth of 'harm reduction'

In the late 1970s and early 1980s, a number of political events dramatically increased the availability of imported heroin in the UK. (Prior to this point, the vast majority of opiates available on the illicit market came from what was termed the 'grey market', diverted legitimate supplies from over-prescribing, pharmacy break-ins, etc.).

Following the revolution in Iran, large numbers of the Iranian bourgeoisie transferred their property into heroin and brought their assets out of the country in that form and the trend continued when the Afghani mujahadeen declared war on the Soviet Union and attempted to drive them out of their country. Much of the funding for this war came from the sale of heroin on the international market. If the 1960s saw an unprecedented rise in the number of young heroin users coming to the attention of treatment services, it was nothing compared with the rise in the early 1980s.

Unlike the previous wave of heroin users who tended to cluster in major cities and often had bohemian tendencies and a subculture that legitimised their drug use, these 'new' heroin users were often working-class or socially excluded, living on council estates all over the place (Pearson, 1987; Parker et al., 1987). Large numbers of them actually had no idea that the drug that they were taking was heroin until they found themselves addicted.

By the middle of the decade, the issue had become a pressing political problem. Parents and local authorities were pressing the government to do something to tackle the issue. Many of these people simply had no idea what had hit them, but when they eventually worked out what it was and tried to send them for treatment, they began to find that there actually was no treatment to send them into. There were no more than a handful of specialist drugs clinics, mostly located in London, and the clutch of voluntary sector services and general psychiatrists running occasional clinical sessions just couldn't cope with the demand for their services. And so in 1985, the Conservative government announced the Central Funding Initiative; a tranche of money from central government that was to be used to make sure that there was a specialist drugs service in every area of the UK.

The second crucial factor that emerged during this period was the identification of HIV and AIDS in injecting drug users (see Chapter 10, this volume). The pressure to do something about the problem grew when epidemiologists working on the problem determined that approximately half of the intravenous (IV) drug users in New York City were HIV positive, and then a young Edinburgh general practitioner named Roy Robinson was doing some tests on a set of blood samples that were taken for hepatitis testing and discovered that some 50 per cent of these blood samples were also HIV positive.

The birth of needle and syringe exchange in Mersey

In response to the Central Funding Initiative, Mersey Regional Health Authority had established Mersey Drug Training and Information Centre (MDTIC), as a resource to provide information to people who were joining this new specialism of drugs work and addiction treatment. In the spring of 1986, some of the staff of MDTIC attended a conference hosted by the World Health Organisation that was convened to discuss the best ways of responding to the threat posed by what was clearly becoming a global pandemic.

Epidemiologists who spoke at the conference were quite clear that the only way that it could be controlled was by preventing the exchange of bodily fluids. This meant the adoption of a number of simple practices. First, everyone who was at risk should use condoms when having sex, and second, the sharing of injecting equipment had to be eradicated.

As an ex-addict himself, one of the delegates from Mersey region, Allan Parry, took the view that the only way that we were going to be able to arrest the spread of HIV in injecting drug users was by supplying them with sterile equipment. However, it was essential if we were to maximise the distribution of equipment among drug users that we do everything possible to remove all obstacles to such a programme's take-up.

In his youth, Allan Parry had a severe addiction problem, and when given the opportunity of going to prison or going to a residential rehab, chose rehab. However, this wasn't just any rehab but a Christian rehab, and after working his way through the programme, Allan eventually ended up as a senior member of staff, before leaving to go to the USA where he worked for the Billy Graham organisation as a lay minister. This unusual background, combined with a naturally charismatic personality, gave Allan a range of important skills that he would draw on effectively in selling the concept of harm reduction over the next few years.

On returning from the conference, Allan lost no time in starting to implement a plan for the first British needle exchange scheme. At the time, this was a highly controversial measure. Most parts of the UK had been working to prevent the distribution of syringes and needles, and in one particular area, the policy had had disastrous effects. Pharmacists in Edinburgh had voluntarily agreed to refuse to supply syringes and needles to anyone other than diabetics or people in possession of a prescription. The equation looked clear. Where the availability of injecting equipment was restricted, such as in Edinburgh and New York, you had rates of HIV infection of around 50 per cent of IV drug-using populations. Where there was free availability of injection equipment, as there had been in Liverpool where injectable prescribing dominated drug treatment, and supplies could be bought from two or three surgical equipment stores in the city centre, HIV infection was non-existent.

These proposals were certainly seen by some as extremely controversial. There were many, many people who believed that supplying injecting equipment to drug users was abdicating a moral responsibility and sending the wrong message. If injecting drug users didn't want to become infected, then they should stop injecting drugs. Others argued that it wouldn't work anyway. Sharing syringes and needles was a central part of the drug subculture, they argued. It was an important ritual, and one that they wouldn't be prepared to give up.

This last point is a classic illustration of how drugs research can provide a completely misleading picture of the patterns of behaviour in drug-using subcultures. Like the ethnographers who have described the sharing ritual, I've also witnessed such behaviour. However, I've only ever witnessed it in quasi-bohemian circles in the early 1970s, among people who were in the very early stages of their drug-using career. Once addiction is established, it's much more common for people to desperately avoid having to wait until after somebody else has had their shot before you have to do your own, and this is particularly true when veins are somewhat damaged and people can take half an hour or longer to successfully complete an injection.

It was clear to us that the people who were citing the sharing ritual as a reason not to do this, were talking from a position of ignorance. We believed that our experience, combined with our reading of the research, meant that we really did know better. Now we had the opportunity to try and prove that to the rest of the world.

Another delegate to the WHO conference was veteran London-based researcher, Gerry Stimson, who was already in preliminary discussions with the government about whether they would support a pilot study to examine the effects of supplying injecting equipment. Although the government agreed to the request, on Merseyside, it was felt that we really couldn't wait for the bureaucracy and had to act as quickly as possible. As it turned out, the government actually acted extremely rapidly, and the Liverpool scheme was established just a few weeks before all of the other pilot schemes in various parts of the UK.

Mersey Regional Health Authority commissioner Howard Seymour also attended the same WHO conference. Seymour was a quiet, scholarly man with entrepreneurial skills and a profound commitment to public health. It was Howard Seymour who had established the Regional Drug Training and Information Centre and persuaded Allan to run it, and he immediately saw the need to act and to act swiftly to establish the needle exchange scheme. Howard approached the Chairman of the Regional Health Authority, Sir Donald Wilson, and rapidly secured his full support for the project, initially to be as an experiment.

In order to avoid running into opposition at the very early stages, Seymour and Parry adopted a very clever strategy. Rather than announcing the scheme, they contacted the local press and told them what they were doing, and impressed upon them the urgency of the task that they faced. They asked the reporter to hold off running the story for two months, after which they'd have an idea whether the project was a success or a failure, and if the latter, they'd close it down.

They also approached the local police at a senior level, and secured an agreement that local officers 'wouldn't hang around outside and target clients'. The officer concerned, Peter Deary, was enormously supportive of the scheme and did a great deal of work, not just to convince his own staff of the value of the project, but also to sell the concept to forces in other areas. Although this may not seem like a major step today, when it seems as though every second officer supports legalisation, the establishment of injecting rooms and wider prescribing of heroin, at that time Peter Deary came in for a great deal of resistance from other forces who criticised the Merseyside Police for having 'gone native' and joined the enemy.

And so a disused toilet cubicle was fitted out with shelves at the Mersey Drug Training and Information Centre on Maryland Street. A nurse was hired, to look at health problems and other difficulties that arose from injecting and to advise clients on technique. The first needle exchange scheme was up and running.

Changes in treatment patterns

At around the same time as the Syringe Exchange Scheme was setting up for business, the new Liverpool Drug Dependency Unit (DDU) opened up.

Throughout the 1970s and 1980s, it was a tenet of faith among some addicts that many, if not all, of their problems would be solved if only the clinics were to return to the practice of heroin maintenance. They would no longer have any need to rely on street drugs, with their impurities and the associated unsterile injection practices. They would no longer be forced to engage in criminal activities in order to maintain their habit, and they would be less inclined to share injecting equipment as they would pick up fresh supplies on a daily basis, along with their medication.

Dr James Willis, the first consultant psychiatrist appointed to run the new DDU, was no stranger to heroin prescribing. He had worked in the London clinics during their early days in the late 1960s and early 1970s (for fuller account, see Chapter 3, volume II). For the last decade or so he had been working in the Middle East, and so had been hidden from the winds of change that had blown through the drugs field over the previous ten years or so. This may explain why he was prepared to initiate a policy of heroin maintenance, when almost nobody else in the UK was prepared to do so. Whatever the reason for his decision, some patients were absolutely delighted and immediately asked that their prescriptions be changed from methadone to heroin.

Unfortunately, for many of this original group, elation rapidly turned to dismay. Used to the long half-life of methadone, they had grown accustomed to using their daily supply all at once, as soon as they picked up their supply. When they tried to do the same thing with diamorphine, they found that their dose just wouldn't hold them until their next pick-up, and so many of them were soon to be seen knocking on the clinic door in withdrawal, asking to be returned to their old regime.

After Dr Willis retired, his position was temporarily filled by Dr John Marks, a general psychiatrist who worked at Halton General and did sessions at drug dependency clinics at Warrington and Widnes.

Two or three years prior to his taking over as acting consultant at the Liverpool DDU, Dr Marks had lectured to my criminology class on his theories about the paradox of prohibition. Methadone maintenance, he argued, was the happy medium between total prohibition and total availability. When he was questioned about the possibility of heroin maintenance, he professed himself in opposition, because of the problems associated with injecting.

By the time he took over at the Liverpool DDU though, he seemed to have overcome his reservations about heroin and rapidly became the most prominent public advocate for a return to the old British System (Marks, 1987, 1995; Eaton et al., 1998), advocating the readoption of both heroin and cocaine prescribing in dosages that are normally regarded as on the high side.

Theorising harm reduction

As a result of these changes in practice and policy on Merseyside, we were well aware that what we were doing constituted a radical break with what was happening throughout the rest of the UK – indeed, throughout the rest of the world. We were aware that we would inevitably come under attack, and so we recognised the need to fortify our defences with good data on the outcomes of our work, and with a theory that underpinned our reasons for doing things the way that we did.

It was Dr Russell Newcombe who came up with the conceptual hook that would provide us with our Trojan Horse. Russell had been working on a prevalence study of drug use on the Wirral, his previous research had been in drug education, and he was about to start a new post in the same area. Russell was much influenced by a project aimed at working with solvent misusers that was produced by researchers at the Institute for the Study of Drug Dependence in the early 1980s.

Drawing on the notion of tertiary prevention, the researchers at the Institute for the Study of Drug Dependence (ISDD) devised an innovative but controversial drugs information project that aimed at teaching those young people who were committed to continued solvent misuse the best ways to minimise any potential harm or from negative consequences.

Whilst not termed as such at the time, this harm reduction initiative resulted in an influential publication that was to remain on ISDD's publication list for a number of years. Four or five years later, Russell had penned an article for *Druglink*, the UK's leading publication for the drugs field, posing the question whether it finally wasn't 'High Time for Harm Reduction' (Newcombe, 1987).

It rapidly became apparent to us that the concept was applicable much more widely than in drug education and prevention, and could actually be used to apply to almost any area of practice or policy. Once the idea had crystallised we set about defining the things that we saw as being the important characteristics of a harm reduction theory (Newcombe, 1992; O'Hare *et al.*, 1992; Heather *et al.*, 1993).

Given that we regarded the existing model of practice and policy as moribund and bankrupt, we gave much of our attention to the characteristics that distinguished harm reduction from the dominant model. For a service or an intervention to be characterised as part of this new paradigm, it should be:

1   *Pragmatic*: recognising that not everybody wanted to, or was able to achieve abstinence. Some people might see it as an eventual goal, others may have no interest in it whatsoever. We took the view that drugs work had to be committed to working with people where they were currently at, not where the worker wanted them to be. At this point, many existing services insisted that their prospective clients had to be committed to abstinence as a goal, and they refused to work with anyone who couldn't demonstrate that commitment.

We took the view that this position was devised to make life easier for the workers, who wouldn't have to sully their hands dealing with the awkward people who still wanted to get high. This was a complete dereliction of duty, in our view. Recovery was a process, and although someone wasn't necessarily ready to give up using at that particular moment, there was still a great deal that could be done in terms of sharing information and building a relationship.

2   *Non-judgemental*: many drugs agencies were often staffed by people with highly judgemental attitudes towards their clients. Why should we care about these people, given they've brought their consequences on themselves by their actions? The people who held these attitudes tended not to have relationships with drug users outside of their work. If they had, they might have realised that every drug user is somebody's son, somebody's daughter. They might have made bad choices, and they often behaved badly from time to time. Nevertheless, if the goal of a service was to engage them, we really had to do everything we could to attract people in. That meant accepting drug users as people. Judge the behaviour, yes, but don't judge the whole person solely because of their problem. Judgemental attitudes on the part of society in general and services in particular were a major reason why most drug users chose not to engage in treatment, and instead to remain in the 'hidden sector'.

3   *User-friendly*: services should actively work towards attracting drug users, working to overcome the obstacles that prevented people using them. This meant locating the premises that were in places that were convenient for large numbers of people to access. Having the entrance in a place that wasn't visible to every passer-by. Opening the project at times when it would get the most use, at times that were convenient to the consumer rather than the worker.

4   *Appropriate*: finally, the services that were provided had to be relevant to drug users' needs. Although some drug users might value in-depth psychotherapy, most thought it was an irrelevance that was conducted for the worker's sense of professional satisfaction and had no bearing on their needs whatsoever. Clean injecting equipment and opiate maintenance were both services that had a high demand, because they made a real and practical difference to people's lives.

These principles sound uncontroversial and obvious today, and so it is hard to convey the sense of radicalism that they engendered in the mid- to late 1980s. At that time, there was an enormous groundswell of opposition to harm reduction from many people who saw this work as explicitly and actively promoting drug use, including strong voices within the drugs field itself for whom the pursuit of abstinence seemed central to their work. So perhaps this opposition wasn't surprising. After all, we were effectively saying to those working in the drugs field that much of what they'd done in the past was completely wrong. And much of what they believed was nonsense. Not only was it not helpful, it was actually an obstacle to change.

As a result, there was a great deal of resistance to our arguments and our strategies. This resistance came from a wide range of interested parties. First, there were the parents, who wanted their children off drugs immediately, and did not consider a maintenance prescription and clean needles to be 'off drugs'. Second, there were the Militant faction associated with the Labour City Council, who had a conspiracy-theory view of the drug problem, which they attributed to Thatcher's attempt to stem the revolutionary potential of working-class youth. Finally, there were some of those working in the field, who resented being told that everything they had ever believed was completely wrong.

Following the huge success of the original syringe exchange scheme, Allan Parry was promoted to Regional Drugs and AIDS Coordinator, and was charged with the expansion of harm reduction policies to services all around the region. Just maintaining our original gains was going to be a tough sell. Expanding those policies outside our local sphere of influence was going to be harder still. Nevertheless, we relished the challenge.

Selling harm reduction to the world

The Regional Health Authority began to implement an expansionist policy, establishing needle exchanges in every area, reducing funding allocations to the old abstinence-oriented 'counselling' services and the very expensive and not very effective rehabs and therapeutic communities.

Where there was resistance, we engaged in hit-and-run guerrilla action research, in which we would recruit a local person who knew the scene, and have them interview local users to get some rough sense of prevalence, of why they did not use services, and of the sorts of risk activities that they engaged in. Armed with this, we would then go back to the service concerned and use the data to strong-arm them into compliance. While this was not the best way to make a lot of friends, it was certainly an effective strategy for getting things done.

Another tool that we employed to our advantage in the furtherance of our mission was the media. Following our success with the local *Echo*, whose original coverage of the needle exchange had been extremely positive, we began to court the national media, but it was not long before courtship was unnecessary. Media coverage of the Mersey Model of Harm Reduction began as a trickle, but over the next few years, was to eventually turn into an avalanche as reporters and television crews began to visit from all over the world to find out exactly what was happening on Merseyside.

A second prong to our ideological offensive began with the *Mersey Drugs Journal* (Matthews, 1987). Initially conceived as a way of keeping the newly recruited class of drugs workers in touch with what was happening in the field, the *MDJ* rapidly started to pick up significant amounts of international subscription. By the end of the first year, the *Journal* had subscribers all over Europe, in Australia and the USA.

It seemed that our challenge to the orthodoxy had touched a chord among large numbers of people, who, prior to this point, lacked a focus for their discontent. The *Mersey Drugs Journal* provided those people with a focus and continued to grow. In 1990, Pat O'Hare took over as director of the Mersey Drug Training and Information Centre, and relaunched the *Mersey Drugs Journal* as the *International Journal on Drug Policy* (Matthews, 1991), and that same year began the International Conference on the Reduction of Drug Related Harm.

Two years after the launch of the needle exchange, we felt that our struggle was officially validated when the Advisory Council on the Misuse of Drugs published its first report on the subject of AIDS and Drug Misuse (1988). Most of our arguments had been enshrined in this document, which we were then able to wave around to further legitimise our mission.

Admittedly, it did not totally support our thesis – it remained ambivalent on the value of heroin and injectable maintenance, accepting only that these have a role in exceptional circumstances. But the report completely supported the need to make and maintain contact with all injecting drug users into services, and was a triumph for the principles of tolerance and pragmatism over more judgemental styles of service delivery and abstentionism; in its most frequently cited conclusion:

> HIV is a greater threat to public and individual health than drug misuse.
>
> (ACMD, 1988)

The decline and fall of the Mersey Model

Unfortunately, what comes up, often also comes down, and the rise of the Mersey Model of Harm Reduction was soon to take a turn in the opposite direction. Perhaps unsurprisingly, the dominance of Merseyside's drugs services by a group of ideological renegades was unlikely to be allowed to continue unchallenged indefinitely. Drug policy and, by extension, drug treatment, is one of the most highly politicised areas of public service provision, and as a consequence, anyone taking a radical position, particularly one that threatens the status quo and challenges the core of a great many people's professional identities, will inevitably find opinion polarised against them.

While some of those responsible for creating and developing this new model of drug service provision on Merseyside in the late 1980s were highly charismatic, not everyone was drawn in by their charisma, and many of those who were initially supportive rapidly began to distance themselves when the tide of opinion turned and certain affiliations began to be regarded as a professional liability.

The downfall began when widespread rumours concerning illicit drug use became prevalent. Not all of these rumours were completely lacking in substance, though even the most accurate tended to be hugely exaggerated, and tended to be spread by people with political motives who lacked any real information or insight into the personal lives of the people concerned, while some of them lacked any connection with reality.

The real problems, in my view, arose not from any unprofessional conduct, but from much more deep-rooted problems that have plagued this field in the past. These included a failure of strategic thinking – a failure to set up systems and structures that would allow the project to continue should any key individuals be removed from or leave their post, for whatever reason.

It must be said though, that certain key individuals exhibited a poor sense of political judgement, a false sense of political invulnerability by some of the individuals concerned, which blinded them to the political realities of the situation in which they found themselves. Rather than consolidating their victories and trying to secure hard evidence for the efficacy of the various radical initiatives that had been established, they went on to announce ever more outrageous developments, often doing so in a time and a manner that was calculated to maximise embarrassment to those that they considered their political enemies.

Two examples of such failures spring immediately to mind. The first was the announcement in one of the tabloids that one of the Merseyside clinics was prescribing cocaine freebase to crack addicts. Even the most ardent anti-prohibitionist and drug policy radical could find little to support such a measure – particularly when it is implemented in such an unregulated manner. I find myself extremely hard-pressed to find any justification for such a practice in the name of addiction treatment; but when you recollect that the practice was announced on the front page of one of Britain's red-top tabloids, on the first day of a Conservative government's conference on demand reduction, a conference which had government ministers from all of the G8 countries in attendance, then the move begins to look positively suicidal in its recklessness.

The second major political embarrassment arose as a result of some of those involved in the Merseyside Harm Reduction Strategy discussing some of the more outlandish local practices on American prime-time television. Rather than presenting these practices as part of an isolated experiment that was gaining popular support, it was claimed that the prescription of large quantities of heroin and cocaine – as much as a gram a day of each, on a take-home basis – was actually mainstream British drug policy, with the implication that this was common practice everywhere. Given the importance of the 'War on Drugs' to the Reagan and Bush administrations, it seems unlikely that questions about these policies were not asked at a very senior diplomatic level, and any goodwill at the national level that may once have existed, rapidly began to dry up.

Of course, as is common in large parts of the public sector and the NHS, nobody was ever actually fired or disciplined for any professional misconduct. However, certain individuals who had previously been central to the debate were eventually sidelined, and job descriptions changed to ensure that they no longer had the sort of responsibilities that would allow them to make such statements in the future.

Due to the way that British drugs services were actually managed at that time, none of the decisions or the public pronouncements that were made could have actually constituted professional misconduct. At that time, clinicians had complete clinical autonomy about how they chose to treat their patients, and senior health service managers enjoyed similar autonomies in terms of determining the sorts of policies and priorities that they would set in their areas. Today, the British System has changed. The Conservative government has established a system of local Drug Action Teams made up of representatives of all the various agencies concerned with local drug problems. New Labour set up the National Treatment Agency whose role is to ensure that treatment services do pursue goals that ultimately have been set by central government. As a consequence, the possibility of another area unilaterally deciding to adopt a strategy for local drug policy that is totally at odds with the rest of the country is now extremely unlikely.

Gains and losses: the Merseyside balance sheet

It is now more than ten years since those who were responsible for establishing the Mersey Model of Harm Reduction left their posts and moved on to other things, and in that time many things have changed. Needle exchange and methadone maintenance are both central aspects of British drug service provision, almost completely non-contentious across most of the UK. The New Labour government has recently declared that cannabis possession should no longer be a policing priority, and Home Secretary David Blunkett has agreed to look at extending the use of heroin maintenance after research in Holland and Switzerland seemed to indicate that it can be a valuable intervention under certain circumstances.

In some senses, then, it could be argued that the progressive agenda that we established on Merseyside in the late 1980s has come to fruition on the national stage. Unfortunately, I would contend that the controversy over harm reduction in the Mersey region has actually had the opposite effect on many of our local services, with a handful of notable exceptions.

In an attempt to avoid any further controversy, services hiring staff tended to look for a safe pair of hands, somebody who was not going to change things, was not going to innovate, and was not going to take risks – a strategy that would have been fine had we been starting from a baseline that already had adequate professional standards of policy and practice. Unfortunately, this just wasn't true. The drugs field in the UK really didn't begin until the mid-1980s, and so much of what passed for practice was actually based on prejudice; what passed for theory owed much more to 'theology'.

Those of us who were responsible for the birth of harm reduction in the UK owed what successes and what insights we had to the fact that we actually *knew* our target groups – they were our friends and, in some cases, we had been part of that group. We knew what would work and what wouldn't. However, when the people at the top changed, those who were to follow dismantled many of the things that worked and worked well, along with some of the things that may have been difficult to justify.

Despite its untimely end, though, the Merseyside experiment had a profound impact on drug policy, not just in the UK, but also on the global stage. As I have already noted, this was not because any of the things that we were saying were particularly new. The libraries were full of books where people discussed these principles in theory. What I believe actually *was* new and radical about what happened back in the late 1980s was that for the first time we had a radical theory that was backed up by actual practice. It was not simply someone saying that this was how you should do it; we were actually doing it, and anyone who was interested could come along and see for themselves whether it worked or not and make up their own mind.

The second thing that I believe contributed to our success was 'branding'. As I have already said, we weren't arguing for anything new, but what we had done was put together arguments from a wide range of disparate sources, and then claimed it as a model that made a radically discontinuous break with existing styles of service provision/ideologies of drug use and drug problems. By stealing the catchy term 'harm reduction' from ISDD, what we had was a new 'high-concept' theory – something that you could pitch to your manager or your funder in a few brief sentences and have them immediately get what was different about this, and the common-sense logic behind it.

By the early 1990s, the UK had totally bought into 'harm reduction' and it was difficult to find somebody working in the drugs field who, regardless of what side of the fence they actually stood on any particular issue, did not describe themselves as being committed to harm reduction – even if what they really meant was that they were diametrically opposed to the same principles that we were committed to.

Conclusions: the future

As with any important social or cultural change, the factors that determine it are often highly contingent on circumstances and accident. Nowhere was this truer than in the role that Liverpool played in the development of the theory and practice of 'harm reduction'.

Had the provision of drugs services been as well developed, centrally planned and directed and professionalised as they are today, the developments of the mid- to late 1980s would almost certainly never have occurred. In many ways, this is a development that should be thoroughly welcomed.

With the rise of new, centralised policy-making institutions, such as the Drug Advisory Teams and the National Treatment Agency, drug policy is becoming ever more determined by government and Whitehall, and drug service provision is becoming more even, and more professional. Hopefully, this means that many of the worst excesses of the past will be ironed out, and we are not yet seeing evidence that this new approach is systematically suppressing innovations or improvements in practice.

Yet at the same time, I cannot help but feel saddened by the fact that the possibility of such a dramatic hijacking of the agenda by a handful of people who lack any real power or status is no longer likely, perhaps even no longer possible.

My account of what happened on Merseyside during that period is inevitably a partial and subjective one. There are others who had greater access to the decision-making processes, and I have no doubt that many of them will disagree with my interpretation of events. Nevertheless, I was one of a handful of people who was actually there at the time, had regular access to all of the key participants, and clearly recognised the fact that what we were doing was, in some small way at least, changing the world.

Despite leading an eventful life, working in drugs research on Merseyside in the 1980s was unquestionably the most exciting time I have ever known. I was working with a group of people who wanted to change that small part of the world that they cared about most, and I believe that we actually succeeded in accomplishing that. Unfortunately, our successes were not anything like as far-reaching as I believe they needed to be, or indeed, as far-reaching as they could have been had we not had a tendency to arrogance and hubris that resulted in a certain degree of self-sabotage.

Much of the discussion contained in this chapter concerns ideological struggles, and fights over mindset and attitude, and it is there that I believe we were most successful. However, those successes should have been backed up by hard evidence. By rigorous and systematic documentation and investigation of the innovations that we initiated back at that time, in this area we failed miserably.

At the First Conference on the Reduction of Drug Related Harm held in Liverpool in 1990, one of the editors of this book, Dr John Strang, said, 'The time has come for the debate around harm reduction to move from something akin to religious dogma to a sounder scientific basis' (later also to appear in the opening chapter in the book from the Melbourne Harm Reduction conference (Strang, 1993). At that time I rejected this statement, viewing it as the last-ditch squeal of a dominant paradigm being overturned, and taking the view that – being grounded in experience and reason – harm reduction was actually much more akin to a well-grounded working hypothesis than a religious dogma.

But any hypothesis needs testing against the real world, not just in clinical practice, but also through rigorous scientific investigation, and on Merseyside we were extremely remiss in our failure to tackle this with the vigour that was necessary. Unfortunately, the statement that I rejected over ten years ago actually seems to have far more validity today, when the fields of drug policy and drug treatment seem to be more polarised than ever before, and many of those professing support for harm reduction include all manner of irrational policies within its remit.

One example that springs to mind is the call for the testing of recreational drugs such as MDMA. Around fifty people a year die as a result of taking MDMA. As far as I am aware, there have been no known deaths that have been a direct consequence of people taking counterfeit tablets, with the exception of a handful of deaths attributed to TMA. Unfortunately, the tests are not sufficiently sensitive to be able to identify the difference between TMA and MDMA, and so these deaths would not have been prevented. One must therefore ask oneself, where is the gain? At best, it creates a false sense of security for the general public and the Establishment from the fact that 'something is being done about the problem'. At worst, by ensuring that people get MDMA rather than a placebo, we actually *increase* the potential for harm rather than actually reducing it.

This kind of irrational thinking seems particularly prevalent in the United States, where the drug legalisation lobby recently stopped organising under the legalisation banner and embraced harm reduction in its place. Over the last few years, I have read articles in harm-reduction journals that have seriously suggested that crack smokers might think about switching to injecting as a harm-reduction measure (McDermott, 2003, and that harm-reduction practitioners have no business being judgemental about needle exchange workers who may occasionally share needles from time to time. It seems to me that the people who make these irrational arguments about issues that seem to me to lie far beyond the remit of harm reduction as a health strategy are all too often recreational drug users who are actually just seeking to justify their own consumption patterns.

I have no problem whatsoever with the argument that the criminal law is an unreasonable method of dealing with drug use and drug addiction, and that criminal sanctions against people for drug use constitute a drug-related harm in themselves. However, there is an important strategic value in a genuine separation between harm reduction as a strategy for improving the health of drug users, and the debate over how successful the criminal law is as a tool for regulating consumption. And I have come to the view that conflating the two issues actually works to the detriment of harm reduction as a public health strategy.

As time passes, many of those who are committed to a reduction of the misery and distress that arises from harmful and damaging patterns of drug consumption are finally beginning to reach a rational *rapprochement* with those we once saw as our enemies. I have finally started to recognise that abstinence-oriented treatment actually does have a useful place, and is something that large numbers of dependent drug users actually seek and are desperate to try and make work for them. The breakthrough, I believe, is the long-overdue recognition that it must not be the sole strategy for dealing with the problem, nor is it in any way superior (and particularly not morally superior) to other strategies that help people effectively address the social and health problems that arise as a consequence of their drug use.

The future, then, must lie not with the continuing polarisation of the debate (harm reduction vs. abstinence-based treatment), but with an attempt to identify areas of consensus about what actually works. Which interventions improve health and a sense of well-being and reduce emotional distress and involvement in criminal activity.

It looks as though the British System is finally figuring out what's needed. Now it's time for the rest of the drugs field to follow suit.

References

Advisory Council on the Misuse of Drugs (1982). *Treatment and Rehabilitation*, HMSO, London.

Advisory Council on the Misuse of Drugs (1984). *Prevention*, HMSO, London.

Advisory Council on the Misuse of Drugs (1988). *AIDS and Drug Misuse, Part 1*. HMSO, London.

Eaton, G., Seymour, H., Mahmood, R. and Marks, J. (1998). The development of services for drug misusers on Mersey. *Drugs: Education, Prevention and Policy*, 5: 305–18.

Fazey, C. (1988). *The Evaluation of Liverpool Drug Dependency Clinic: The First Two Years 1985–1987*. Research Evaluation and Data Analysis, Liverpool.

Heather, N., Wodak, A., Nadelman, E. and O'Hare, P. (eds) (1993). *Harm Reduction: From Faith to Science*. Whurr Publishers, London.

McDermott, P. (2003). Crack harm reduction doesn't wash. *Druglink*, 18(4): 20.

Marks, J. (1987). State-rationed drugs. *Druglink*, 2(4): 15.

Marks, J. (1995). Who killed the British System? *Druglink*, 10(4): 3–4.

Matthews, A. (ed.) (1987). Editorial, *The Mersey Drugs Journal*, 1(1). Liverpool.

Matthews, A. (ed.) (1991). Editorial, *The International Journal on Drug Policy*, 1(1). Liverpool.

Mitcheson, M. (1994). Drug clinics in the 1970s. In Strang, J. and Gossop, M. (eds) *Heroin Addiction and Drug Policy: The British System*. Oxford University Press, Oxford.

Newcombe, R. (1987). High time for harm reduction. *Druglink*, 2(1): 10–11.

Newcombe, R. (1992). The reduction of drug-related harm: a conceptual framework for theory, practice and research. In O'Hare, P., Newcombe, R., Matthews, A., Buning, E. and Drucker, E. (eds) *The Reduction of Drug Related Harm*. Routledge, London.

O'Hare, P., Newcombe, R., Matthews, A., Buning, E. and Drucker, E. (eds) (1992). *The Reduction of Drug Related Harm*. Routledge, London.

Parker, H., Newcombe, R. and Bakx, K. (1987). *Living with Heroin: The Impact of a Drug Epidemic on an English Community*. Open University Press, Milton Keynes.

Pearson, G. (1987). *The New Heroin Users*. Blackwell, Oxford.

Self, W. (1992). Drug dealer by appointment to H.M. Government. *The Observer*, 13 September 1992.

Seymour, H. and Ashton, J. (1990). *The New Public Health*. Routledge, London.

Spear, B. (1994). The early years of the British System in practice. In Strang, J. and Gossop, M. (eds) *Heroin Addiction and Drug Policy: The British System*. Oxford University Press, Oxford.

Stimson, G. (1994). Minimizing Harm from Drug Use. In Strang, J. and Gossop, M. (eds) *Heroin Addiction and Drug Policy: The British System*. Oxford University Press, Oxford.

Stimson, G. V. and Lart, R. (1991). HIV, drugs and public health in England: new words, old tunes. *The International Journal of the Addictions*, 26: 1263–7.

Strang, J. (1993). Drug use and harm reduction: responding to the challenge. In Heather, N., Wodak, A., Nadelman, E. and O'Hare, P. (eds) *Harm Reduction: From Faith to Science*. Whurr Publishers, London.

Chapter 12

Different types of heroin in the UK

What significance and what relationship to different routes of administration?

John Strang, Paul Griffiths and Michael Gossop

(This chapter draws substantially on material originally published in journal form as: Strang, J., Griffiths, P. and Gossop, M. (1997) Heroin in the United Kingdom: different forms, different origins, and the relationship to different routes of administration. *Drug and Alcohol Review*, 16: 329–337, supplemented by material taken from the paper by John Strang and colleagues (2001) on 'Different forms of heroin and their relationship to cook-up techniques: data on, and explanation of, use of lemon juice and other acids'. *Substance Use and Misuse*, 36: 573–587.)

Heroin is often assumed to be a constant product, apart from variation in the purity of the black market products or the contaminants. Through the last quarter of the twentieth century in the UK, this has increasingly become a mistaken, and dangerous, assumption.

Prior to the 1960s, this presumption of a constant product was well-founded. Virtually all heroin in the minute British heroin 'scene' was pharmaceutical heroin (diamorphine hydrochloride) in the form usually of the tablets ('jacks') or occasionally in the powder form of diamorphine hydrochloride BP. The former was available on the black market as a result of diversion from supplies prescribed to heroin addict patients or as a result of chemist burglaries, whilst the latter, rarer, product was almost exclusively as a result of burglaries. Descriptions of these early days can be found within the various accounts written both contemporarily and subsequently (Second Brain Report, 1965; Spear, 1969; Spear, Chapter 3, this volume). Thereafter, there has been considerable variety to the products in the heroin marketplace.

Pharmaceutical heroin has become a much smaller part of the black market but is still available, although almost entirely in the form of freeze-dried ampoules of heroin – mostly as diversion of supplies prescribed to a small number of heroin addict patients. However, by the 1980s and thereafter, most heroin on the black market was imported heroin, usually imported from South East or South West Asia (O'Neil *et al.*, 1984; Billiet *et al.*, 1986).

Heroin purities

Purity of black market heroin in the UK has varied little over the last decade, (even though price in real terms has dropped steadily), and the mean purity of samples analysed from street seizures during each three-month period of the last two decades is shown in Figure 12.1.

Drug purities are calculated by the UK Forensic Science Services as the proportion of heroin base in the sample, and not as the proportion of any particular salt (see later within this chapter). Heroin samples analysed by the Forensic Science Services are obtained from Police seizures in the UK (often termed street seizures, so as to emphasise the difference from Customs seizures). The mean purity of seizures for any quarter has always been between 20 and 50 per cent during the last decade, and the distribution of purity of individual samples (from which the mean for each quarter is calculated) is scattered across the full purity range but with an approximately normal distribution: in the samples analysed during the first quarter of 1994, for example, nearly half of all seizures fell in the range 20–50 per cent (212 of 433 samples; 49 per cent), with 82 samples (19 per cent) below this range and 139 samples (32 per cent) above this range. Figure 12.1 also shows the typical price per gram of a street sample of this black market heroin – both as the actual price per gram, and also as price corrected for each year according to changes in the cost-of-living index.

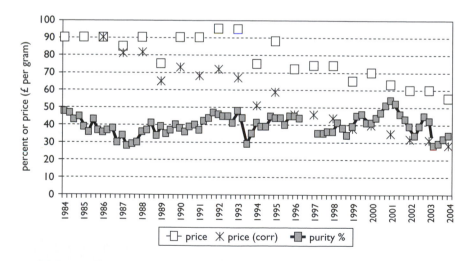

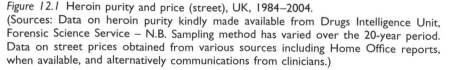

Figure 12.1 Heroin purity and price (street), UK, 1984–2004.
(Sources: Data on heroin purity kindly made available from Drugs Intelligence Unit, Forensic Science Service – N.B. Sampling method has varied over the 20-year period. Data on street prices obtained from various sources including Home Office reports, when available, and alternatively communications from clinicians.)

Whilst domestic law enforcement agents and treatment personnel pay little attention to the different types of heroin, heroin users themselves often pay great attention to these different products in the marketplace, pay different sums for different forms, and use the different heroins often by different routes.

Brown and white heroin: is there any significance to the distinction?

White forms of heroin are, in general, more sought after and are believed by heroin users themselves to be substantially higher purity heroin (Lewis *et al.*, 1985). There is no evidence of any significant continuation of the market in 'Marseilles heroin' from the network of heroin laboratories in Southern France which had been so dominant from the early 1950s (Vaille and Bailleul, 1953) up until the early 1970s (McCoy, 1972; Galante and Sapin, 1982). This network of laboratories involved refinement of the bulkier opium and morphine concentrates which were brought to France from Turkey and South East Asia for Marseilles conversion into a high-purity white heroin hydrochloride (Lamour and Lamberti, 1974; Auger, 1978). The breaking of the 'French Connection' in 1972/73 coincided with, or was followed closely by, a change in the manufacture of heroin, with transfer of the technology to sites much closer to the production fields. Since the mid-1970s, heroin has been produced in laboratories near to the harvest areas and has hence been shipped usually in the form of (less bulky) heroin (Hartnoll *et al.*, 1984; Lewis, 1985).

The first substantial amounts of imported black market heroin in the UK were forms of heroin known as 'Chinese Heroin' or other names indicating its South East Asian origin (e.g. Hong Kong rocks) (Spear, 1975) which, in the late 1960s and early 1970s, were typically purchased from dealers in the Chinese community in or around Gerrard Street in Soho, London (Ashton, 1982; Lewis, 1985). The two main forms were Heroin No. 3 and, more usually, Heroin No. 4.

Heroin No. 4 is often pure white or slightly off-white, and is a light powdery heroin of high purity – often as high as 90 per cent (O'Neil *et al.*, 1985). It is recognised as being of higher quality, may be known as 'No. 4' or by other names such as 'Thai Heroin' or 'White Elephant', and commands a higher price on the black market. It is always injected.

Heroin No. 3 is typically somewhat granular and varies in colour between mid-brown and dirty off-white (O'Neil *et al.*, 1985). It is usually of lower purity than Heroin No. 4 with both active and inactive diluents – some being other psychoactive drugs such as 6-mono-acetyl-morphine, morphine and acetyl codeine, whilst other components merely add bulk (such as sugars). Strychnine has sometimes been found in low concentrations in heroin, but the amounts have been far below a level at which any discernible effect would result, and the rationale behind the inclusion of strychnine in the manufacture has remained unclear (Eskes and Brown, 1975). Heroin No. 3 has been used both for smoking/chasing the dragon, and also for injecting.

During the late 1970s and early 1980s, it became clear that samples of black market heroin were being 'cut' with (altered by the addition of) barbiturates (O'Neil et al., 1984), and this was often presumed to be an attempt by dealers involved in further adulteration of the heroin who were seeking to mimic the psychoactive effect of the heroin. However, an alternative explanation is that, at some stage in the production procedure, there may have been an awareness that the addition of barbiturates increases the recovery (i.e. the amount of heroin the user actually receives as a dose) from use of the heroin by smoking (Gruhzit, 1958; Huizer, 1987; Billiet et al., 1986).

In general, these were the only forms of illicitly-manufactured heroin which were to be found in the UK until the late 1970s, apart from occasional appearance of small quantities of other South East Asian heroins such as 'Hong Kong rocks' and 'Red Chicken'. These South East Asian heroins (No. 3 and No. 4) were virtually always in the form of the hydrochloride (diamorphine hydrochloride).

South West Asian brown heroins began to appear in the UK during the second half of the 1970s. Lewis (1985a, 1985b) identifies 1978 and 1979 as the watershed years, with this new form of brown heroin entering Europe in the wake of the Iranian revolution; O'Neil et al. (1984) report on the change in samples of heroin sent for forensic analysis at this time in the UK, with a similar change at this time reported by Huizer (1987). This brown heroin was introduced alongside the spread of the new form of heroin use by 'chasing the dragon'. In the subsequent 15 years, South West Asian heroin has established and retained a dominant position in the black-marketplace, albeit with moves between different forms of South West Asian heroin (Iranian, Turkish, Pakistani, etc.) – so much so that by 1994 the Forensic Science Service at Aldermaston commented specifically on an unusual seizure of white heroin, stating: 'Unlike the brown South West Asian product, white heroin (probably from South East Asia) has not been seen in the UK for many years' (Forensic Science Service, 1994).

It is not entirely clear how drug users establish whether or not these different brown heroins are, or are not, suitable for injection or smoking. Heroin users report that all brown heroins can be used by chasing the dragon, and that white heroins are particularly suitable (and almost always purchased for) injecting. However, brown heroins are also sometimes injected even though, as Lewis observed: 'Dark brown smoking heroin, although often containing a high opiate content, was crudely refined: such heroin often causes problems when prepared for injection' (Lewis, 1985).

Table 12.1 Heroin recovery rates after 'chasing the dragon'

Compound	Recovery (%)
Heroin hydrochloride	17%
Heroin hydrochloride + caffeine (1 + 1)	36%
Heroin hydrochloride + caffeine (1 + 4)	51%
Heroin hydrochloride + barbital (1 + 1)	33%
Heroin hydrochloride & procaine hydrochloride (1 + 1)	12%
Heroin (base)	62%
Heroin (base) + caffeine (1 + 1)	76%

Source: Huizer (1988)

Heroin samples in the form of the hydrochloride or the base

The diamorphine in samples of black market heroin in the UK is sometimes in the traditional form of the hydrochloride, and on other occasions is in the form of heroin base. Neither heroin users nor drug workers nor policy makers appear aware of this difference in the form in which the heroin is available. This is surprising as the difference in form has clear implications for the different main routes by which the heroin is likely to be used: heroin in the hydrochloride form is typically injected, whereas heroin base is particularly suitable for chasing the dragon. Some, and perhaps even all, forms of heroin base can be converted into the hydrochloride by the addition of, for example, citric acid or some other acid, and may form part of the reason for the emergence of the use of citric acid powder, vitamin C powder, Jif lemon juice or vinegar as agents used in the 'cooking up' process of preparation of heroin for injection.

The importance of the form of the heroin (as a salt or in the base form) and the presence of different diluents or cutting agents has recently been explored by Huizer (1987). Huizer attempted to reconstruct in the laboratory the heating of heroin on tinfoil so as to simulate chasing the dragon. He found major variations in the recovery of heroin after minor changes to the way in which the heroin was heated – similar to the variation described by heroin users themselves. Huizer then went on to examine heroin recovery from different forms of heroin (base and salt) and forms of this heroin mixed with caffeine, with barbiturate, and with procaine: recovery of heroin as a proportion of the heroin in the original sample in Huizer's study is shown in Table 12.1.

Subsequently Huizer examined the impacts on heroin recovery during simulated chasing the dragon with one-to-one mixtures of heroin base (the most widely available form of black market heroin in Europe during the

1980s) with a variety of different possible fillers or cutting agents. This showed further significant effects on the recovery of both heroin and monoacetyl-morphine, with virtual elimination of heroin recovery after the addition of ascorbic acid. In contrast, the addition of methaqualone (formerly available in the UK in the drug Mandrax, and still available as illicitly imported supplies from the Continent) resulted in a high recovery of heroin at 55 per cent. The latter observation may explain the discovery of barbiturate or methaqualone as 'contaminant' in some samples of black market heroin used by heroin addicts in the UK (Sanger *et al.*, 1979; O'Neil *et al.*, 1984).

White heroins would seem always to comprise heroin in the hydrochloride form – hence marketed for and suitable for injection. Brown heroins, on the other hand, may be in the form of the hydrochloride or the base. Indian heroins, for example, have typically been processed more rigorously prior to the acetylation during the black market refinement of the morphine base, and are consequently of a higher purity and in the form of the hydrochloride. Of all seizures of Indian heroin by UK Customs in the four years up to 1982, all but two of the samples were in the form of the hydrochloride with the remaining two being in the form of the free base (O'Neil *et al.*, 1984). In contrast, after the brief appearance of South West Asian heroin in the hydrochloride form in the late 1970s, all seizures of Iranian heroin made by UK Customs in the four years up to 1983 were of the form of heroin base, except for one single seizure of the hydrochloride, and the samples of heroin base additionally contained caffeine, and sometimes also barbiturates, which would have rendered the heroin particularly suitable for chasing the dragon (O'Neil *et al.*, 1984). The heroin content of these South West Asian heroins was usually intermediate between the purities for South East Asian No. 3 and No. 4, and in the UK the purity of street heroins has been reasonably constant over the last decade at somewhere between 25 and 45 per cent (see Figure 12.1 again).

The UK Forensic Science Service has brought together the findings from their different laboratories on different cutting agents/adulterants used in heroin seizures, and have reported internally on their survey of cutting agents used in a random sample of 228 seizures of heroin examined in UK laboratories in 1995/96 (unpublished data, Forensic Science Service, 1996). Only two cutting agents were commonly found – paracetamol in 33 per cent of samples and caffeine in 32 per cent of samples, whilst no cutting agent was found in 44 per cent (inorganic compounds, and sugars such as manitol and glucose, were excluded from the analyses, although frequently used as bulk inert fillers during cutting of black market heroin samples). From Huizer's studies (see above) caffeine would lead to increased recovery of the heroin during chasing the dragon when using either the salt or base form of heroin. The influence of the paracetamol is not so clear; its main influence may be to increase the recovery of one of the first degradation products of heroin – 6-mono-acetylmorphine (6-MAM) – which is recovered in substantially

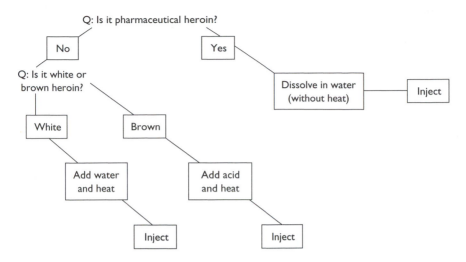

Q: Is it pharmaceutical heroin?

No

Yes

Q: Is it white or brown heroin?

Dissolve in water (without heat)

Inject

White

Brown

Add water and heat

Add acid and heat

Inject

Inject

Figure 12.2 The decision to inject heroin
Source: Strang *et al.* (2001).

greater proportions after the 'chasing' of heroin/paracetamol mixtures (Huizer, 1988).

Different preparation techniques and conversions between different forms of heroin

From the late 1970s onwards, it has become common practice for injecting heroin users to incorporate simple chemistry – the addition of acid – into the preparation of their black market heroin to ensure appropriate solubility of the illicitly produced sample of heroin. In particular, this has applied to the increasing availability of base forms of heroin (i.e. not the salt form), which, without specific preparation, are not reliably suitable for injection. This detail of the preparation of heroin was investigated and reported by Strang *et al.* (2001), and the following is a summary of these findings. The necessary preparation of their heroin typically involves the addition of an acid in the form of either vitamin C, or citric acid. Other forms of acid such as vinegar or lemon juice are also used on rare occasions. Typically this also involves the application of heat to the mixture of the illicit heroin powder and the acid, in order to obtain a solution of the heroin which is considered suitably prepared for injection. On the basis of the findings from interviews with current heroin users, it was possible to construct a 'virtual' decision-making algorithm which describes how the relevant decisions were made as to whether to include or omit acid and heat to the process of preparation of the heroin for injection – see Figure 12.2.

Bio-availability of heroin and breakdown products with 'chasing the dragon'

Study of the extent of absorption of heroin by smoking was commissioned by the League of Nations in the 1930s and was studied by Ito (1937), who reported that no active components were contained within the smoke when heroin was burnt (Bulletin on Narcotics, 1953). However, 'chasing the dragon' and the preceding 'smoking' of heroin pills both involved techniques which did not burn the heroin, but rather heated it to a temperature at which sublimation would occur. In a study of the bio-availability of heroin by different routes, Mo and Way (1966) examined the total morphine recovery from urine from subjects taking measured doses of heroin by smoking in cigarettes, by chasing the dragon and by intravenous injection. They found morphine recovery rates of 14 per cent, 25 per cent and 68 per cent, respectively, for a given dose of heroin, thus indicating an approximate bio-availability of 20 per cent and 40 per cent for the smoking of heroin in cigarettes and in chasing the dragon. Cooke and Brine (1985) later studied the pyrolysis products of heroin – both in the salt form (diamorphine hydrochloride) and as heroin base. The three major pyrolysis products in the 250°C pyrolysate were 6-O-acetylmorphine, N,6-O-diacetylnormorphine, and N,3-O,6-O-triacetylnormorphine – with the same pyrolysis products occurring with heating of either the salt or the base (Cooke and Jeffcoat, 1990). Huizer followed the earlier work from Cooke and Brine with a study of the effects of heroin in a variety of conditions simulating chasing the dragon and with the heroin in salt and base form and in the presence of various diluents (summarised earlier in this chapter). In addition to altering the total recovery of heroin and morphine, the addition of diluents also altered the proportions of the different pyrolytic products. When heroin base was heated on aluminium foil, there was a resulting higher overall heroin bio-availability compared with when the heroin hydrochloride was heated, and, amongst the pyrolytic products, monoacetylmorphine predominated. The addition of caffeine increased the heroin recovery and was associated with an increased monoacetylmorphine recovery, in much the same way as had been described by Mo and Way (1966) in their studies of the effect of the addition of daii fan (barbiturate) to heroin in chasing the dragon.

Country of origin and the form of the heroin

Several reports on the arrival or spread of heroin in a community have included reference to both the type of heroin and the country of origin. Thus Leong (1980) describes the arrival of heroin No. 3 from Thailand: furthermore he identified that the heroin No. 3 was only suitable for use by smoking in cigarettes or by chasing the dragon, and was unsuitable for injecting. Similarly, reports on heroin use in the Netherlands (Huizer et al., 1977) and in the UK (Lewis et al., 1985) include descriptions of the types and countries of origin of the different forms of heroin. However, such accounts are based entirely on the self-report of the study sample themselves.

Identification of the country of origin of seized quantities of black market heroin has developed over the years with advances in laboratory study of the physical form and analytical techniques. Such an approach was already used in the years after the Second World War (Bulletin on Narcotics, 1953) in which the distinction was made that, in addition to estimating the actual diamorphine content of black market heroin, it was possible to consider the various other components as either diluents (often sugars or some other inert bulk), adulterants (other drugs such as quinine or barbiturate which themselves have actions), impurities of manufacture (such as monoacetylmorphine and morphine, resulting from imperfect acetylation in the black market laboratory), and impurities of origin (such as meconic acid and other brown colouring matter which indicate a crude production process in the original morphine extraction), or the use of morphines with different ratios of the various alkaloids. At this time, these adulterants and impurities of manufacture and origin were already studied, their variation over time recorded, and it was already possible for a series of samples of black market heroin in New York to be identified as from the same source in the eastern Mediterranean (Bulletin on Narcotics, 1953).

With the development of improved gas-chromatographic techniques and mass spectrometry (Twitchett, 1975; Van der Slooten and Van der Helm, 1975; Moore, 1978) and the use of high performance liquid chromotography (HPLC) (Baker and Gough, 1981; Chow et al., 1983), it has been possible to improve the accuracy of study of the 'fingerprint' of the different forms of black market heroin (Billiet et al., 1986). This improvement in technology enabled laboratory identification of the country of manufacture of seized samples of heroin No. 3 and heroin No. 4 which were the two forms of heroin described by Huizer et al. (1977) from the Netherlands, and Neumann and Gloger (1982) and O'Neil et al. (1984, 1985) in the UK have subsequently identified the fingerprints of the various forms of heroin from different parts of the world. All types of heroin from the global marketplace have been identified in seizures in the United Kingdom with the exception of Mexican heroin which appears to be directed entirely towards North America (O'Neil et al., 1985). The heroin preparations from different countries, therefore, exist in different physical and chemical forms, and are thus of differing suitability for either smoking or injecting. In their review of the different forms of black market heroin in the late 1970s and early 1980s, O'Neil and his colleagues at the Home Office Forensic Laboratory identified the following types of heroin appearing in different chemical forms (O'Neil et al., 1984, 1985):

1 *Heroins of Pakistani origin*: these varied considerably in both colour and consistency, ranging from light to dark brown, and, whilst usually a fine

powder, had occasionally been seized in the form of small aggregates. Typical purity was in the 70–80 per cent range. Whilst seizures during the 1970s had been in the form of diamorphine hydrochloride, all recent seizures had been in the form of the base, with the exception of one particular white fine Pakistani heroin of even higher purity which was present in the hydrochloride form.

2   *Heroin from Iran*: this form of heroin was physically and chemically similar to heroin from Pakistan, although with less variation in physical appearance and chemical form, and was found in all but two instances to be in the form of heroin base.

3   *Heroin from Turkey*: this light brown heroin was always in fine powder form and was present as the hydrochloride salt.

4   *Heroin from South East Asia*: various South East Asian heroins were seized including 'Chinese No. 3' (a granular heroin varying in colour from grey to brown), 'Chinese No. 4' the sought-after fine white powder, and the less frequently encountered 'Penang Pink', a granular heroin similar to Chinese No. 3 but dark pink in colour. Chinese No. 4 was always found to be in the salt form (diamorphine hydrochloride) whilst the other two forms were found sometimes as salt and sometimes as free base.

5   *Heroin from India*: Indian heroin was a white fine powder similar to Chinese No. 4 and always in the salt form (diamorphine hydrochloride).

Seizures of heroins with other countries of origin (including Lebanon, Syria and Nigeria) were rare, and were always found to be in the salt form (diamorphine hydrochloride).

Conclusion

Heroin in the UK (and across most of Europe) now exists in a variety of different forms – in the salt or base form, and with the presence or absence of other drugs. These make a substantial difference to the suitability for use by different routes. In particular, the recovery rates on using samples of heroin by 'chasing the dragon' vary according to its base or salt format and according to the presence of other drugs in the sample, with the presence of caffeine doubling or tripling the heroin recovery (varying with the exact ratios), and the addition of barbiturates doubling recovery, and with heating the base form giving a yield more than three times greater than the heating of an equivalent amount of heroin hydrochloride. Attention to the different types and forms of heroin needs to become a routine part of clinical, customs and criminal enquiry as well as being part of the trading and purchase patterns of heroin users themselves.

References

Ashton, M. (1982). What's happening with heroin? *Druglink*, 17: 1–5.
Auger, M. (1978). *The heroin triangle*. London: Methuen.

Auld, J., Dorn, N. and South, N. (1986). Irregular work, irregular pleasures: heroin in the 1980s. In Mathews, R. and Young, J. (eds) *Confronting Crime*, pp. 167–187. London: Sage.

Baker, P. J. and Gough, T. A. (1981). The separation and quantitation of the narcotic components of illicit heroin using Reversed Phase High Performance Liquid Chromatography. *Journal of Chromatographic Science*, 19: 483–489.

Billiet, H. A. H., Wolters, R., De Galan, L. and Huizer, H. (1986). Separation and identification of illicit heroin samples by liquid chromatography using an alumina and C_{18} coupled column system and photodiode array detection. *Journal of Chromatography*, 368: 351–361.

Bulletin on Narcotics (1953). The mysterious heroin pills for smoking. *Bulletin of Narcotics*, 5: 54–59.

Bulletin on Narcotics (1953). History of heroin. *Bulletin on Narcotics*, 5: 3–16.

Bulletin on Narcotics (1953). The analysis of heroin. *Bulletin on Narcotics*, 5: 27–38.

Bulletin on Narcotics (1958). Chasing the dragon: the smoking of heroin in Hong Kong. *Bulletin on Narcotics*, 10: 6–7.

Chow, S.-T., O'Neil, P. J., Baker, P. J. and Gough, T. A. (1983). A comparison of chromatographic methods for the estimation of the diacetyl morphine content of illicit heroin. *Journal of Chromatographic Science*, 21: 551–554.

Cooke, C. E. and Brine, D. R. (1985). Pyrolysis products of heroin. *Journal of Forensic Sciences*, 30: 251–261.

Cooke, C. E. and Jeffcoat, A. R. (1990). Pyrolytic degradation of heroin, phenocyclidine and cocaine: identification of products and some observations on their metabolism. In Chiang, C. N. and Hawks, R. L. (eds) *Research findings on smoking of abused substances* (NIDA Research Monograph No. 99), pp. 97–120. Rockville, Maryland: National Institute on Drug Abuse.

Eskes, D. and Brown, J. K. (1975). Heroin–caffeine–strychnine mixtures – where and why? *Bulletin on Narcotics*, 27: 67–69.

Forensic Science Service (1996). Unpublished report.

Galante, P. and Sapin, L. (1982). *The Marseilles Mafia*. London: Allen Lane.

Gamella, J. F. (1994). The spread of intravenous drug use and AIDS in a neighbourhood in Spain. *Medical Anthropology Quarterly*, 8: 131–160.

Gruhzit, C. C. (1958). Pharmacological investigation and evaluation of the effects of combined barbiturate and heroin inhalation by addicts. *Bulletin on Narcotics*, 10: 8–11.

Grund, J.-P. and Blanken, P. (1993). *From chasing the dragon to Chinezen: the diffusion of heroin smoking in the Netherlands*. Institut voor Verslavingson der Zoek (IVO Series 3). Rotterdam: Erasmus University.

Hartnoll, R., Lewis, R. and Bryer, S. (1984). Recent trends in drug use in Britain. *Druglink*, 19: 22–24.

Huizer, H. (1983). Analytical studies on illicit heroin: No. 2 comparison of samples. *Journal of Forensic Sciences*, 28: 44–48.

Huizer, H. (1987). Analytical studies on illicit heroin: 5-efficacy of volatilisation during heroin smoking. *Pharmaceutisch Weekblad*, Scientific Edition, 9: 203–211.

Huizer, H. (1988). Efficacy of volatilisation during heroin smoking. *Analytical Studies for Illicit Heroin*, pp. 107–126. Netherlands: Ministry of Justice.

Huizer, H., Logtenberg, H. and Steenstra, A. J. (1977). Heroin in the Netherlands. *Bulletin on Narcotics*, 29: 65–74.

Ito, R. (1937). Amount of effective component which passes into smoke when heroin is smoked. (Original Japanese Abstract described by Cooke, 1991).

Lamour, C. and Lamberti, M. (1974). *The second opium war*. London: Allen Lane.

Leong, J. H. K. (1980). Beating the gong and chasing the dragon in the Lion City. *Journal of Drug Issues*, 10: 229–240.

Lewis, R. (1984). The illicit traffic in heroin: Introduction and Part 1 – cultivation and production. *DrugLink*, 19: 7–14.

Lewis, R. (1985). Serious business – the global heroin economy. In Henman, A., Lewis, R. and Malyon, T. (eds) *Big deal: the politics of the illicit drugs business*, pp. 5–49. London: Pluto.

Lewis, R., Hartnoll, R., Bryer, S., Daviaud, E. and Mitcheson, M. (1985). Scoring smack: the illicit heroin market in London, 1980–1983. *British Journal of Addiction*, 80: 281–290.

McCoy, A. W. (1972). *The politics of heroin in South East Asia*. New York: Harper & Row.

Mo, B. P. and Way, E. L. (1966). Assessment of inhalation as a mode of administration of heroin by addicts. *Journal of Pharmacology and Experimental Therapeutics*, 154: 142–151.

Moore, J. M. (1978). Rapid and sensitive gas chromatographic quantitation of morphine, codeine and O^6-acetyl morphine in illicit heroin using an Electron Capture Detector. *Journal of Chromatography*, 147: 327–336.

Neumann, H. and Gloger, M. (1982). Profiling of illicit heroin samples by High-Resolution Capillary Gas Chromatography for forensic application. *Chromatographia*, 16: 261–264.

O'Neil, P. J., Baker, P. B. and Gough, T. A. (1984). Illicitly imported heroin products: some physical and chemical features indicative of their origin. *Journal of Forensic Sciences*, 29: 885–902.

O'Neil, P. J., Phillips, G. F. and Gough, T. A. (1985). The detection and characterisation of controlled drugs imported into the United Kingdom. *Bulletin on Narcotics*, 36: 17–33.

Oldendorf, W. (1992). Some relationships between addiction and drug delivery to the brain. In Frankenheim, J. and Brown, R. (eds) *Bioavailability of drugs to the brain and the blood-brain barrier* (Research Monograph 120), pp. 13–25. Rockville, Maryland: National Institute of Drug Abuse.

Oldendorf, W. H., Hyman, S., Braun, L. and Oldendorf, S. Z. (1972). Blood-brain barrier: penetration of morphine, codeine, heroin, and methadone after corotid injection. *Science*, 178: 984–986.

Sanger, D. G., Humphreys, I. J. and Joyce, J. R. (1979). A review of analytical methods for the comparison and characterisation of illicit drugs. *Journal of Forensic Science Society*, 19: 65–71.

Spear, H. B. (1969). The growth of heroin addiction in the United Kingdom. *British Journal of Addiction*, 64: 245–255.

Spear, H. B. (1975). The British experience. *The John Marshall Journal of Practice and Procedure*, 9: 67–98.

Strang, J. and King, L. (1996). Heroin is more than just diamorphine (editorial). *Addiction Research*, 5: 3–7.

Strang, J., Gossop, M., Griffiths, P. and Farrell, M. (1989). The technology of dragon chasing. *British Journal of Addiction*, 84: 669.

Strang, J., Des Jarlais, D. C., Griffiths, P. and Gossop, M. (1992). The study of transitions in the route of drug use: the route from one route to another. *British Journal of Addiction*, 87: 473–484.

Strang, J., Griffiths, P., Powis, B. and Gossop, M. (1992). First use of heroin: changes in route of administration over time. *British Medical Journal*, 304: 1222–1223.

Strang, J., Griffiths, P. and Gossop, M. (1997). Heroin in the UK: different forms, different origins, and the relationship to different routes of administration. *Drug and Alcohol Review*, 16: 329–337.

Strang, J., Keaney, F., Butterworth, G., Noble, A. and Best, D. (2001). Different forms of heroin and their relationship to cook-up techniques: data on, and explanation of, use of lemon juice and other acids. *Substance Use and Misuse*, 36: 573–587.

Vaille, C. and Bailleul, E. (1953). Clandestine heroin laboratories. *Bulletin on Narcotics*, 5: 1–6.

Van der Slooten, E. P. J. and Van der Helm, H. J. (1975). Analysis of heroin in relation to illicit drug traffic. *Forensic Science*, 6: 83–88.

Chapter 13

Use of illegal drugs in Northern Ireland

The strange case of a surprisingly small problem

Diana Patterson

Introduction

Northern Ireland is a region with much stress from civil unrest and economic disadvantage. One might expect high levels of misuse of heroin and other drugs but this is not the case. Heroin use is low, running at about 10 per cent of the rate of misuse in other parts of the UK. This low use also contrasts with the high rate of misuse in some other parts of Ireland, notably Dublin. The size of the problem and factors influencing heroin use are examined in this chapter.

Size of the problem

There is surprisingly little heroin use in Northern Ireland, and surprisingly little drug injecting behaviour. The Addicts Index Notification procedure has survived in Northern Ireland because of its small size and clinical usefulness. In 1997, 162 notifications were made to the Northern Ireland Addicts' Index for a population of 1,600,000. Of these, 120 notifications were for opiate misuse, 78 of which were for heroin. The Index does not include those addicted to dihydrocodeine or codeine. The number of people registered on the Northern Ireland Addicts' Index has risen gradually from 51 in 1991, to 60, 80, 87, 96, 120 and 162 over the next six years. This rate constitutes approximately 10 per cent of the rate of misuse of opiates in other parts of the UK and contrasts with high rates of heroin misuse in Southern Ireland where 3,839 individuals were treated for opiate misuse in a population of 3,500,000 in 1996 (Moran *et al.*, 1996). In stark contrast, a substantial Irish injecting opiate misuse problem occurred around the Dublin area, growing progressively from the early 1980s onwards, and yet Dublin is only 110 miles by road from Belfast and the other main population centres in Northern Ireland.

Population surveys give us an indication of the level of drug misuse in Northern Ireland. The Health Promotion Agency for Northern Ireland has carried out studies in 1992 and 1994 on the health behaviour of school children (Health Promotion Agency for Northern Ireland, 1995). In the 1992 study, among 15 year olds, 25.2 per cent said they had been offered drugs at least once. Sixteen per cent of the sample of 804 children had tried drugs or solvents and 6 per cent were currently using drugs. Cannabis was the most frequently used drug. Heroin did not show up in this survey. The survey was repeated in 1994. Twenty-six per cent of 15 year olds had used drugs or solvents from a sample of 1,150 children, and 42 per cent of these had been offered drugs. In this study 3,932 children were studied from three age bands: 11 years, 13 years and 15 years. Five children claimed to have used heroin. This constituted 0.1 per cent of the sample. The findings from these studies suggest rates of drug misuse lower than those from comparable studies in the UK. Millar and Plant (1996) reported findings from different regions of the UK. The region reported to have the lowest level of drug misuse was Northern Ireland with 25.6 per cent reporting that they had used any drug. The absolute number of individuals who identify heroin as a drug they have used is very small in all of these surveys.

The Northern Ireland Crime Survey was carried out between October 1994 and January 1995. This was described by Boyle and Morgan (1997). This was a household survey of 2,200 people where respondents were encouraged to answer questions honestly about drug use by taking control of the keyboard to answer without oversight by the interviewer. Seventeen per cent of the sample admitted ever taking at least one of the listed drugs. Cannabis, amphetamines, LSD, magic mushrooms, amyl nitrate, tranquillisers and ecstasy were the most commonly used drugs. Use of heroin and methadone was negligible. Cocaine was misused by only 0.2 per cent of the sample. Another household study also described by Boyle and Morgan (1997), the Northern Ireland Omnibus Study, carried a drugs module in September 1996. Over 813 people agreed to take part. There was a general increase in drug use with 28 per cent of the sample now admitting use of a drug at some time, but no increase was noted in the use of heroin or methadone which remained negligible. This was repeated in September 1997 and described by the Northern Ireland Office (1998) with 969 responders, when 24 per cent of the sample admitted use of a drug at some time. In both surveys the most commonly used drug at any time in the past was cannabis. In 1996, 20 per cent of the population surveyed stated that they had used cannabis and this figure was reduced to 16 per cent of the survey sample in 1997. The 1997 survey continued to show negligible rates of use of 'hard' drugs such as crack, heroin, cocaine or methadone. In the 1997 study, 27 per cent of males and 20 per cent of females admitted ever using any drugs. There was a statistically significant decrease in the percentage of males who stated that they had ever used a drug from 37 per cent in 1996 to 27 per cent in 1997, but no significant reduction in the percentage of females using drugs. Sample sizes were relatively small and the drug-using population is known to be difficult to reach through household surveys. In all other sample surveys in the Province all forms of drug use have shown a gradual increase over time. The Addicts' Index shows a slow rise of 10 per cent to 30 per cent each year over the last six years.

Drug-injecting behaviour has not been a traditional part of the drug culture in Northern Ireland. Although drugs such as amphetamines and dihydrocodeine are widely reported as misused, these drugs do not seem to be injected to any significant extent. An audit was carried out in April 1997 of all patients presenting to the statutory Addiction (drug and alcohol) Treatment Centre in Belfast, with a catchment population of 360,000, over the preceding 12 months. Twenty-eight of the 225 patients presenting with drug misuse, stated that they had ever injected any drug. Thirteen of those were still using intravenous heroin at the time of presentation. All of those patients reported using heroin and several reported injecting other drugs, most notably amphetamines. Fifty-four per cent of this group reported that their injecting behaviour had begun within Northern Ireland, the remainder having begun their injecting behaviour outside the Province.

Of the statutory notifications made to the Chief Medical Officer in Northern Ireland during 1997, 68 patients were reported to have injected at some stage in their lives (DHSS (NI), 1997). This was a slight increase on earlier years.

It can, of course, be argued that a much larger problem may exist than is recognised in terms of both heroin use and injecting drug misuse. It might be, for example, that people using heroin do not present to the treatment services as methadone maintenance is not offered as a treatment. However, the physicians and surgeons and doctors from the Accident and Emergency Departments do not report treating sequelae of drug-injecting behaviour such as abscess or limb ischaemia. The spread of HIV and hepatitis C in the Province through drug misuse appears to be low. By October 1998 526 individuals had demonstrated antibodies to the hepatitis C virus in Northern Ireland. Testing had commenced for hepatitis C at the Regional Viral Laboratory in 1992. Only 45 individuals over this time had their hepatitis C antibodies attributed to intravenous drug misuse. In total, 175 individuals in Northern Ireland had a positive reaction to the polymerase chain reaction. Fourteen of these individuals had their active viral activity attributed to drug misuse.

Information from the Royal Ulster Constabulary (Northern Ireland Office, 1998) suggests that recorded drug offences have increased by 61 per cent in Northern Ireland over the past five years, from 620 in 1992 to 998 in 1997. Over the same period there has been almost a 50 per cent increase in drug arrests. Drugs seized by the Royal Ulster Constabulary during 1997 included 111,851 tablets of LSD, 78,108 tablets of ecstasy, 24 kilograms of amphetamine, 486 kilograms of cannabis, 426 grams of cocaine and 196.5 grams of heroin. All drug seizures show increases of magnitude of at least 400 per cent since 1992 with considerable variation year on year as figures can be distorted by single seizures.

Factors predisposing to drug use

Let us reflect on some of the reasons why we might expect a high level of misuse of heroin within Northern Ireland. Large sections of the population are disadvantaged both socially and economically.

The population has been exposed to substantial stress through civil unrest. 'The Troubles' in Northern Ireland started in 1966 and by December 1997 3,585 people had been killed (Bloomfield, 1998) as a direct result of the troubles with more than 40,000 people injured in civil unrest (Social Services Inspectorate, DHSS (NI), 1998) out of a population of 1.6 million. Many more people had been intimidated and forced to leave their homes or places of work. Substantial numbers of people have carried on their lives with a very real risk of death or serious injury from paramilitary organisations. Others have been forced to leave the Province under threat. An IRA cease-fire in September 1994 followed by a Loyalist cease-fire in October 1994 gave comparative 'peace' for a time. 'Punishment beatings' and murders continued during this time as paramilitary groups sought to 'police' and retain control over their own districts and populations. This cease-fire ended with the Canary Wharf bombing in London in February 1996.

The 'Good Friday Agreement' of 10 April 1998 was reached by the Governments of Great Britain and the Republic of Ireland, and by the major political parties of Northern Ireland. The Agreement was strongly supported by a census of the population in Northern Ireland on 22 May 1998. While the peace process put in train to bring political stability to the region has suffered a number of set backs, it is clear that, at present, there is a strong desire by the large majority of the population in Northern Ireland to work towards peace.

There are good road and rail communications between Northern Ireland and the Republic of Ireland. Several heroin users in Belfast report travelling to Dublin on a frequent basis by road or by train to buy heroin for their own use. Some also report using these routes as couriers, bringing in larger supplies for other individuals.

Travel between Northern Ireland and the mainland United Kingdom is also straightforward. There are major haulage ferry routes operating from Stranraer and Cairnryan in Scotland to Larne, a port in the North East of Northern Ireland. Regular ferries also sail between Belfast and Liverpool. There are regular flights from two airports in Belfast to several major cities in England, Scotland and Wales. The postal services act as an import source for several drugs of misuse including heroin.

Ireland, as an island, has traditionally been an exporter of people, although this tendency has decreased over time. Large numbers of well-educated young people leave Northern Ireland each year, some to attend universities on the UK mainland. Some of these young people return to the Province in later years. Some people enter Northern Ireland in order to obtain work. It is rather surprising that, despite the civil strife, over recent years there has been a net immigration to Northern Ireland. One might expect that this two-way flow of population would result in eventual import of heroin or the population who might use the drug.

Factors protecting against heroin misuse

Factors directly related to the civil unrest

One obvious result of the civil unrest is a high level of security in the Province. In particular, the scrutiny at the land and sea borders by Customs and Excise Officers has been intense. Although the scrutiny has been directed in the past to the movement of arms, ammunition and explosives, there is no doubt that it has discouraged straightforward importation of both large and small amounts of the illicit drugs. The high Police presence, the number of roadblocks and personal searches has also discouraged the selling of drugs on the street. There has been significant monitoring of personal movement of citizens by the Security Forces, particularly around the border areas. Again this has tended to discourage the free movement of drugs.

Paramilitary organisations on both sides of the sectarian divide have made threats to shoot and kill 'drug dealers'. Such threats have been carried out and serious gunshot injuries have been inflicted on several people in the Province who have known histories of drug misuse. Several individuals have been murdered, apparently because of drug misuse or drug dealing. Many individuals have left the Province, often at very short notice after threats have been made to them that they would be shot. However, it is interesting that this form of paramilitary control has not stopped the import of cannabis, ecstasy, LSD or amphetamines. The rave scene in Northern Ireland developed in 1991 and the increase in these drugs has been steady and inexorable since that time. Several paramilitary organisations are believed to have benefited financially from international drug dealing but all have maintained a strong 'anti-drugs stance' within Northern Ireland. This very real deterrent has probably been the single largest factor in dissuading people whose origins lie outside Northern Ireland from attempting to bring drugs into the Province.

The environment in Northern Ireland, particularly in urban areas, is off-putting to drug users. The sight of armoured cars and heavily armed police and army personnel is not conducive to the drug-taking attitudes and lifestyle. Those who take drugs and who are attracted by the drug-taking lifestyle may find the environment unattractive and may be inclined to leave.

The parochial nature of Northern Ireland

Communities in Northern Ireland tend to have good social cohesion. Most children still live with two biological parents. The churches and schools still have an important place in the communities they serve. The parochial nature of the environment may help to protect children from drug taking.

Anti-social behaviour, including drug taking, is less likely to be ignored than it is in other environments where this level of social cohesion does not exist.

Strength of the RUC Drug Squad

The RUC Drug Squad was formed well before there was any major drug problem in Northern Ireland. It came into being at the same time as the Drug Squads in other parts of the UK and at a time when drug problems were emerging in the UK. The Drug Squad has traditionally had a high level of intelligence and has always been relatively well manned. A strong preventive Police response to drugs was thus provided before the drug problem became insurmountable. The size of the Drug Squad was effectively doubled in 1996 by the then Chief Constable of the Royal Ulster Constabulary, Sir Hugh Annesley.

Medical response

There is a voluntary ban on out-patient methadone prescribing by all doctors in Northern Ireland. This is rather similar to the voluntary ban on barbiturate prescribing in the 1970s. The only opiate drugs substantially misused in the community at present are dihydrocodeine and codeine. These are not notifiable drugs and therefore there are no hard data on the levels of misuse. The levels of dihydrocodeine prescribing are on a par with those in other parts of the UK. The reluctance to prescribe maintenance methadone arises from the dangers of diversion. Small amounts of methadone prescribed to out-patients have been stolen by paramilitaries, presumably for sale. There are very real fears of increasing the pool of opiates available on the black market in Northern Ireland.

The medical response to those addicted to opiate drugs is normally to offer withdrawal. Methadone is used for opiate withdrawal, usually on an in-patient hospital basis. Beds for detoxification from heroin can usually be offered within a few days of presentation. More recently lofexidine has been used extensively by the statutory services to alleviate symptoms of withdrawal. The advantage of this medication is that it can be offered to patients who are prepared to attend hospital daily as day-patients. Approximately 50 per cent of heroin withdrawals are now managed in this way. The majority of the remainder are detoxified as in-patient cases using a mixture of lofexidine and methadone. This treatment appears to be very acceptable to patients.

This response, of course, results in part in export of methadone users. Some individuals approach services in Northern Ireland for continuation of maintenance scripts which they have received in the UK or other countries. When they are offered detoxification but not maintenance methadone they may choose to leave the Province. Doctors in Northern Ireland may thus be accused of 'exporting the problem'.

Against this must be weighed the fact that many people come to Northern Ireland in order to obtain a drug-free environment when they have decided to withdraw from heroin. There is recognition that they will receive help with withdrawal, and that it is difficult to obtain supplies of heroin and methadone at street level in Northern Ireland.

The price of peace

Since 1991, there has been a steady increase in the use of all illicit drugs in Northern Ireland. 'Peace' was first considered a reality in 1994 with the sustained IRA and Loyalist cease-fires. The popular press, at that time, began to pay attention to the increase in the level of drug misuse. There were prophecies that the cease-fires would lead to relaxation of the paramilitary response in preventing drug misuse and there was talk of an 'explosion' in drug use in Northern Ireland. In fact, the rate of increase in heroin use, injecting and other drug use has risen steadily and does not appear to have been affected by the cease-fires of 1994, the resumption of hostilities in 1996, or by the Good Friday Agreement of April 1998. Sadly, it is likely that, over time, as the borders within Europe become less noticeable, that the level of drug use within Northern Ireland will increase to match that of its neighbours.

References

Boyle, M. and Morgan, S. (1997). Changing Patterns of Drug Use in Northern Ireland – Some Recent Survey Findings. Northern Ireland Office – Research Findings.

Bloomfield, Sir Kenneth, KCB (April 1998). Report of the Northern Ireland Victims Commissioner. We Will Remember Them. The Stationery Office, Northern Ireland.

DHSS (NI) (31 December 1997). Northern Ireland Drug Addicts' Statistical Information Bulletin.

Health Promotion Agency for Northern Ireland (1995). The Health Behaviour of School Children in Northern Ireland (HBSC). A Report on the 1994 Survey. World Health Organisation Collaborative Study.

Miller, P. and Plant, M. (1996). Drinking, Smoking, and Illicit Drug Use among 15 and 16 year olds in the United Kingdom. *British Medical Journal*, 313: 394–397.

Moran, R., O'Brien, M., Duff, P. (1996). Treated Drug Misuse in Ireland. National Report. The Health Research Board.

Northern Ireland Office (November 1998). Patterns of Drug Use in Northern Ireland – Some Recent Survey Findings: 1996–1997. NIO – Research Findings, 2/98.

Social Services Inspectorate, DHSS (NI) (March 1998). Living with the Trauma of the 'Troubles'. Report.

Chapter 14

The relationship between the state and local practice in the development of national policy on drugs between 1920 and 1990

Gerry V. Stimson and Rachel Lart

(This chapter originally appeared in J. Strang and M. Gossop (eds) *Heroin Addiction and Drug Policy: The British System*, Oxford University Press, 1994.)

There never was such a thing as the 'British System' for dealing with drug problems. There was never a 'system' in that there was no grand idea, no grand plan, and no systematic practice. Instead, there was a loose and shifting collection of ideas and practices, at times appearing firm and definite, becoming elusive on closer examination. It was not 'British', because although policy documents and legislation applied throughout the United Kingdom, this hid a distinctive and growing national and regional diversity.

What was distinctive was not the overall plan, the idea or the practices, so much as the relationship between the state in the form of central government, and the various professions and groups which have claimed an interest in drug problems. What came to be called the 'British System' was really a reflection of the way social and health policy emerged within the United Kingdom. As such, we have to understand drugs policy, not as an entity in its own right, but as part of the broader trends in social policy.

From the 1920s to the 1960s

The 'British System' was created by its commentators. The term was coined by E. W. Adams, who had served as secretary to the Rolleston Committee and helped draft its report in 1926 (Adams 1937). But in the United Kingdom, we really discovered that we had a 'system', when our approach to drug problems became useful ammunition for protagonists in the United States. Between the late 1940s and the early 1960s, they strongly argued against the criminalization of addiction and looked favourably at the supposed medicalization of drug addiction in the United Kingdom. A series of UK watchers and visitors, including Rufus King (1972), Alfred Lindesmith (1965) and

Edwin Schur (1963), thought that we did things better. In essence they argued that we had only a minor problem with the major drugs of abuse such as heroin and cocaine, because our addiction problems had been contained within a system of medical treatment. We were justly proud and flattered by their comments and complacently and inaccurately agreed with their wisdom.

Their, and our, interpretations exaggerated the significance of the report of the Rolleston Committee, which had legitimized the medical treatment of addiction (Departmental Committee on Morphine and Heroin Addiction 1926). The Rolleston Committee considered that it was appropriate, in certain circumstances, for doctors to prescribe drugs of addiction to those addicted to them. The Rolleston Committee Report set the scene for the next 40 years, and remained the only point of reference for those seeking to understand the formal underpinnings of our approach. There was no other document to read: this is not to suggest that many in fact read it. There is a certain irony that sociological commentators from the United States argued for the benefits of the medicalization of drugs problems, when a few years later other sociological commentators would argue so strongly against medical dominance.

There is a second irony in that the description of the 'British System' as primarily a medical (and hence, many would claim, benign) approach, was only a partial description of United Kingdom policy. As Berridge has pointed out, the medical response to drug problems always operated within a penal and legal framework (1984). Since the 1920 Dangerous Drugs Act, we could, and did, send people to prison for the unauthorized possession of dangerous drugs. However, many commentators on the 'British System', in focusing on the medical involvement, rarely gave much attention to the penal response.

The approach outlined by Rolleston was class-based. It was designed for the respectable and deserving addict. It was geared to the therapeutic addict – the iatrogenic victim – whose addiction was an accidental side-effect of medical treatment, and to the 'professional' addict, which was official euphemism for doctors, nurses and veterinary surgeons who had become addicted through raiding their drugs cabinet or writing false prescriptions.

The medical approach outlined by Rolleston began to fall apart during the 1960s with the emergence of the unrespectable and undeserving addict, who had started to use drugs for fun and excitement, and who continued for self-gratification. Hedonistic drug use did not fit easily into the image of drug addict as victim of medical practice or of occupational hazard.

The policy disintegrated in face of the rising numbers of youthful heroin and cocaine users in the 1960s (Stimson and Oppenheimer 1982). Forty years after Rolleston, it was time to look again at British Drugs Policy. Of the two reports produced by the Brain Committee in the 1960s, the second was the new landmark (Interdepartmental Committee on Drug Addiction 1965). The Brain Committee did not abandon a medical approach to the treatment of drug addiction, but argued that there were some flaws in allow-ing general medical practitioners to prescribe heroin and cocaine to people addicted to these drugs. Whilst general practitioners may have been willing to treat the respectable addict, only a handful would take on the youthful heroin addict. Some of those who did were dedicated and deserved the respect of their colleagues who shunned this work; others were of more doubtful motivation and judgement, and quite clearly some were being conned by their patients.

The problem for the Brain Committee was how to maintain medical interest but introduce some control over medical practice. This it did by taking the treatment of addiction out of the hands of the general practitioner, and into the hands of, for the most part, psychiatrists. This 'psychiatrization' of the problem fitted well with the growth of psychiatry in the 1960s.

On paper this was still a medical approach. The caveat as always, was the continuing role of the penal and legal system. But medicine remained centre stage by dominating the discourse on the nature of drug problems. Just as in the 1920s, the experts of the 1960s were doctors.

Distinctive features of the medical involvement in drug problems

Both US and UK commentators pointed to the significance of a medical involvement. For some it was a particular medical practice that was import-ant, specifically the ability to prescribe drugs such as heroin to addicts. This was not – and is still not – allowed in many countries. Trebach (1982) indicated how matter-of-factly the British medical profession was allowed to use a drug which invited horror and condemnation in the United States. It has always been possible for any medical practitioner to prescribe heroin in the treatment of normal medical conditions (and is still so today). Although prescribing heroin to addicts was a British claim to fame, such prescribing was all but over by about 1970. The major period of prescribing heroin was in the 1960s and during the first couple of years of the drug dependency clinics which had been established post-Brain in 1968. From then on methad-one was the drug of choice.

For other commentators it was not prescribing *per se* that was important, but a distinctive relationship between doctor and patient. Rather than being required to treat all addict patients the same way, the British medical practi-tioner could use his or her discretion in the kind of treatment offered. Patients were treated as individuals, rather than slotted into an inflexible programme. It is indicative in this period that the United Kingdom did not have treatment 'programmes', and that there was little administrative and legal guidance on the treatment of addiction. Contrast this with the United States, where methadone programmes were subject to compendious regulation.

Commentators who pointed to the relationship between doctor and patient were perhaps more accurate in their assessment than those who pointed to the actual practices. Any visitor to a British Drug Dependency Clinic would have been bewildered by the array of treatment regimens and the inability of the consultant to describe the treatment approach in simple terms. Eclecticism and pragmatism ruled the day. The other side of the coin was that in this flexible situation, no one would force a medical practitioner to prescribe for addicts. As a result there were parts of the country where there was no prescribing.

Drug policy, the state and the medical profession

This special relationship with the patient is the clue to understanding what was distinctive about the approach to drug problems in this period. It was not that doctors were able to prescribe heroin, but the fact that they had the choice to do so or not.

The medical approach to drug problems resulted from an accommodation between the state and a powerful profession. The claim that the medical profession made to be free from control by the state or by patients, and to be a self-regulating occupational body, meant that as an occupation it had extremely high levels of autonomy. In the tussle between the state's desire to do something about the drug problem, and the medical profession's desire to retain its power, clinical freedom emerged unscathed. It was doctors who were called on as experts on their own behalf in the 1920s and again in the 1960s and to give judgement on legitimate medical practice, and later to produce guidelines for good medical practice.

That this was the case in the 1920s should not be surprising, given the dominance of private medical practice. It might seem surprising in the post-1948 nationalized National Health Service (NHS), where there would appear to be more opportunity for central regulation over clinical activity.

However, this was not the case until very recently. Up to the introduction of general management in 1984–85, there was no real mechanism for central control of peripheral activity within the NHS. Indeed, such mechanisms were explicitly rejected at the start, with Bevan's view that the NHS was there to provide the framework which would leave doctors free to do their work. The only means of regulation that central government had was that of overall budgetary control. Prior to the 1974 reorganization, management was conspicuous by its absence; administrators' and treasurers' roles were to administer and keep financial order, not to take a proactive line in the development of services. Clinical autonomy, the medical practitioner's right to exercise his or her professional judgement in the choice of treatment for any individual patient was not only protected within the NHS, but enhanced by the removal of concern over the immediate financial consequences of decisions. Professional judgement meant the application of medically accepted knowledge, but left a wide margin for individual variation in practices and techniques. What actually happened within the NHS was the sum total of individual consultants' decisions, rather than a result of defined policy aims.

The period of consensus management following the 1974 reorganization of the NHS tended to reinforce rather than curb this medical dominance, with the real locus of power frequently being outside the management team and in the hands of individual clinicians (Royal Commission on the National Health Service 1978). It was only in the mid-1980s that there was a serious attempt, with the introduction of the Griffiths-style general managers, to shift the frontier of control between central government and the medical profession.

In the field of addiction, this emphasis on clinical autonomy allowed for the variety of treatments (including no treatment at all) through the whole period from the 1920s through to the late 1960s. There was no Department of Health or Home Office policy-making body to plan a British strategy. The Home Office Drugs Branch played an important behind-the-scenes role from the 1930s and had powers under various dangerous drugs legislation to call aberrant doctors to order, but in practice it rarely invoked formal sanctions, preferring instead, a gentlemanly British nod and a wink.

Policy making in this period was done by calling together committees of 'the great and the good'. At times of crisis, the unpaid volunteer professional class was called on to make judgements and steer the country in the right direction. The period is marked by ad hoc committees – first Rolleston and later Brain. There was no politicization of drugs problems, indeed in true gentlemanly British fashion, politics were excluded from debate.

Jeffery Weeks, in discussing the wider social reconstruction of morality that went on in the 1950s and 1960s, illustrates this with a comparison of the debates over issues such as homosexuality and abortion in the United States and Britain. In the United States the debate was politicized and employed the language of rights and of appeals to justice within the framework of a defined constitution. In this the state had a role in positively affirming an individual's rights. In Britain the debate was about privacy; defining the boundaries between private and public behaviour, and limiting the state's interference. The US style demanded 'drama and national campaigns', while the British style was one of 'delicate manoeuvring, parliamentary persuasion and political stealth' (Weeks 1985), an essentially private world where policy was made by accommodation between experts and civil servants.

The establishment of the Advisory Council on the Misuse of Drugs (ACMD) in 1971 continued in this vein. Although meeting on an ongoing basis rather than convened in response to crises, its composition reflected that tradition of British Committee membership and its debate was characterized by a lack of politics and an ethic of politeness. The fact that it was an 'Advisory' committee also indicates the loose British approach to policy making. The Advisory Committee could advise, but Ministers did not have to listen.

The first conclusion is that drugs policy emerged from a particular relationship between the state and the medical profession. What has been identified *vis-à-vis* the medical profession and drugs reflected more generally the relationship between the State and the medical profession and thus what was possible in medicine in Britain. It also reflected, as is argued below, particular relations between the centre and periphery in social and health policy.

Drug policy in the 1980s

There were several changes in policy and practice in the period from the beginning of the 1980s. The first significant feature was the decline in centrality of medicine in the response to drug problems, in comparison with earlier times. Drug Dependency Clinics and the medical treatment of drug problems continued, but there was a shift in balance and doctors no longer dominated the discourse on drug problems (Stimson 1987).

Throughout the 1980s there was the growth of new drugs agencies, funded under the Central Funding Initiative. In fact, the majority of drugs agencies started work from the mid-1980s onwards (MacGregor *et al.* 1991). As indicated elsewhere (Stimson and Lart 1991; also see Chapter 16, this volume) this resulted in many new occupational groups being drawn into working with drug users, freed to some extent from preoccupations with medical treatment and abstinence. The multiplicity and diversity of institutional sites enabled the rapid development of a new discourse on drug problems, which came to be seen as 'harm minimization'. Although much of the medical work done from the 1920s could also be described as harm minimization, it was not so described at the time. This concept is a key to understanding a new way of viewing drug problems and dealing with drug users.

The multiplicity of institutional sites, and the prevailing discourse on harm minimization, were important precursors to the response to the acquired immune deficiency syndrome (AIDS) and the human immunodeficiency virus (HIV) (Stimson and Lart 1991). In the period from 1986 when AIDS became a prominent issue, many drugs agencies were able to respond readily and rapidly to the problem (Stimson 1990). The willingness to discuss and adopt many new strategies – such as syringe distribution and syringe exchange, new ways of working with methadone, a hierarchy of objectives, and innovative educational approaches – could only have emerged given these pre-conditions. It is significant that much of what came to be considered commonplace in the current British response to AIDS and drugs misuse was considered anathema in the United States. It would not be possible for a government committee in the United States to make a statement such as those made by the ACMD, and to retain its credibility. The guiding statement from ACMD was that AIDS was much more of a threat to individual and public health than drugs (ACMD 1988).

Drug policy, the state and the new drugs strategy

There was considerable flexibility in response to HIV and AIDS, much innovation and adaptability to local circumstances. At first sight, this might seem to be a repetition of the story of professional autonomy and practical freedom. Indeed, the 1980s allowed for a high level of freedom for workers in these new agencies. However, we would suggest that this has to be understood in terms of the new relationship between the state and health and social welfare in the 1980s. There was a new balance between central direction and local activity. The new situation reflected the ideas of marketplace Thatcherism, coupled with a claim to non-interference at a local level in order to encourage local accountability. The claimed demise of the 'nanny state' in fact hid a new, and perhaps stronger, form of centralism which operated mainly through control of resources.

This balance, made up of new and complex central/peripheral relations, has been noted by several commentators. In the early 1980s the emphasis was on devolving responsibility for managerial decisions, as outlined in the policy document *Care in Action* (Department of Health and Social Security (DHSS) 1981), and exemplified by the abolition of the Area Health Authority tier of management and the creation of the District Health Authorities. Smaller and smaller units were to make more decisions about implementation of policy. Allsop (1984) commented that 'the strategy is to diffuse responsibility for policy change to the periphery', while Parston (1988), more positively, noted a 'sense of local determination' on the part of the new Health Authorities. The NHS was no longer a monolithic structure with uniform patterns of administration, but demonstrated local variations. For example, with the implementation of the Griffiths' Management Inquiry, each District was free to determine its own structure and pattern of units and management. This period, the early 1980s, was one of fragmentation.

Following this, there was the development of a new kind of centralism. The District Health Authorities and then the Griffiths' general managers were supposed to be close enough to local services and local needs to make decisions in a way that was sensitive to local variations and conditions. However, the pressures of financial constraints and the use of controlling techniques such as individual performance review and performance-related pay tended to make management more upward than outward looking. Devolved responsibility turned out in practice to mean increased accountability, and particularly financial accountability. There was also a growing tendency for central government to tell the periphery how to carry out this 'devolved responsibility' by the issuing of guidelines, directives and circulars. An American commentator noted this trend, describing how, over a six-week period, the paper thus distributed to each District amounted to a stack eight inches high (Light 1990).

This new relationship between the central state and local practice in health care had three elements. First, the power of medicine was challenged and the extent to which the medical profession would act as *de facto* policy makers was curtailed. Second, the unified structure of the NHS was broken and, below District level, structures and power relations varied, resulting in diversity and a degree of local autonomy. Finally, the state found more sophisticated ways to exert central control than its former method of overall budgetary limits; the issuing of directives and exhortations, coupled with tighter mechanisms of accountability. In the drugs field these three elements unravelled in particular ways.

First, as noted above, there was the displacement from centre stage of a purely medical perspective on drug use and the drug user. Second, fragmentation and local diversity in service provision were especially characteristic of drug services. The nearest thing to national plans for service provision were the various reports of the Advisory Council on the Misuse of Drugs (ACMD 1982, 1984, 1988, 1989) and the health circulars following them which, in true British style, 'drew attention to' their recommendations.

Linked to this was a third element: increased centralism. In the drugs field this was exemplified by the fact that the government began to play an active role in drugs policy making and drugs strategy. This could be seen in the establishment of the Ministerial Group on the Misuse of Drugs, an inter-ministerial committee with representatives from all government departments who had some interest in the drugs problem. It was only under the Conservative administration that a British government has produced a strategy document on tackling drug misuse. Prior to this period, there were no formal planning mechanisms. It was also found in the funding mechanisms, such as the Central Funding Initiative, and the earmarked allocation of money given for AIDS and drugs. In both, the approach was to encourage local activity by the allocation of resources, coupled with a central but brief statement about the desirability and nature of certain services, but then with a lack of oversight and control over the actual nature and day-to-day work of those services.

This centralism in drugs services and policy did not, yet, involve the financial constraints that constituted its coercive element elsewhere in health services. While services could have operated better and reached more clients if they had had more money, it has also to be acknowledged that drug services did, in the 1980s, receive unprecedented levels of finance. The nature of that finance is crucial to this discussion. It was delivered in the form of the Central Funding Initiative and, since 1986, earmarked allocations. The use of these was intended to reinforce the view that drug services were regarded at central level as a national priority; money for them was to be protected from the local politics of allocation. In the wider view then, finance for drug services reflected the increasing centralism within health policy. At the level of practice, the diverse nature of services as they developed reflected the lack of central control over day-to-day work and procedures.

Thus, the setting for the new drugs policy was a particular social policy framework that allowed for strong central direction accompanied by local autonomy. How this balance between central control and local activity was to be affected by the next stage of NHS reforms from 1990 onwards must form part of a further analysis.

In conclusion

It is not the particular ideas and practices which are the key to understanding the British response to drugs, so much as the framework in which these ideas and practices are allowed to emerge.

For much of the time from the 1920s through to the 1980s drugs policy was shaped by a particular relationship between the state and medicine. The general high levels of autonomy accorded to the medical profession in this period allowed doctors to hold centre stage as experts on addiction, to define drug problems in medical terms (as some kind of disease), and allowed them to choose suitable treatments. In the 1980s, drugs policy was shaped by the new relations that developed between the state and medical and social services, with robust central influence, accompanied by an emphasis on local expertise and decision making.

Future students should cease to abstract drugs policy from the wider stream of British social policy and the structures in which that policy is produced. Policy about and services for drug users are not a special arena with a unique set of relations between central government and Health Authorities, professions and agencies in the field. The nature and style of relations between the state and the medical profession, and of central/peripheral relations would appear familiar, if somewhat exaggerated, to many general commentators on the NHS.

References

ACMD (Advisory Council on the Misuse of Drugs) (1982). *Treatment and rehabilitation*. Report. HMSO, London.

ACMD (1984). *Prevention*. Report. HMSO, London.

ACMD (1988). *AIDS and drug misuse. Part 1*. Report. HMSO, London.

ACMD (1989). *AIDS and drug misuse. Part 2*. Report. HMSO, London.

Adams, E. W. (1937). *Drug addiction*. Oxford University Press, London.

Allsop, J. (1984). *Health policy and the National Health Service*. Longman, London.

Berridge, V. (1984). Drugs and social policy: the establishment of drug control in Britain 1900–1930. *British Journal of Addiction*, 79, 17–29.

Departmental Committee on Morphine and Heroin Addiction (1926). Report. (The Rolleston Report.) HMSO, London.

DHSS (1981). *Care in action*. HMSO, London.

Interdepartmental Committee on Drug Addiction (1961). Report. (First Brain Report.) HMSO, London.

Interdepartmental Committee on Drug Addiction (1965). Second report. (Second Brain Report.) HMSO, London.

King, R. (1972). *The drug hang-up: America's fifty-year folly*. Norton, New York.

Light, D. (1990). Biting hard on the research bit. *Health Service Journal*, 25 October, 1604–5.

Lindesmith, A. R. (1965). *The addict and the law*. Indiana University Press, London.

MacGregor, S., Ettorre, B., Coomber, R., Crosier, A. and Lodge, H. (1991). *Drug services in England and the impact of the Central Funding Initiative*. Report. Institute for the Study of Drug Dependence, London.

Parston, G. (1988). Evolution – general management. In *Reshaping the National Health Service* (ed. R. Maxwell). Policy Journals, Berkshire.

Royal Commission on the National Health Service (1978). *Research Paper No. 2: Management of financial resources in the National Health Service*. HMSO, London.

Schur, E. M. (1963). *Narcotic addiction in Britain and America*. Tavistock, London.

Stimson, G. V. (1987). British drug policies in the 1980s: a preliminary analysis and suggestions for research. *British Journal of Addiction*, 82, 477–88.

Stimson, G. V. (1990). AIDS and HIV: the challenge for British drug services (Fourth Thomas James Okey Lecture). *British Journal of Addiction*, 85, 3, 329–39.

Stimson, G. V. and Lart, R. A. (1991). HIV, drugs and public health in England: new words, old tunes. *International Journal of the Addictions*, 26 (12), 1263–77.

Stimson, G. V. and Oppenheimer, E. (1982). *Heroin addiction, treatment and control in Britain*. Tavistock, London.

Trebach, A. S. (1982). *The heroin solution*. Yale University Press, New Haven.

Weeks, J. (1985). *Sexuality and its discontents*. Routledge & Kegan Paul, London.

Chapter 15

The development of the voluntary sector

No further need for pioneers?

David Turner

(This chapter originally appeared in J. Strang and M. Gossop (eds) *Heroin Addiction and Drug Policy; The British System*, Oxford University Press, 1994.)

The British response to emerging drug problems was remarkably similar to the response to any other social problem. Having determined that there was no problem one year (HMSO 1961), a couple of years later the same Committee (Interdepartment Committee on Drug Addiction: The Brain Committee) was hastily being reconvened to make recommendations on how to respond to the problem which had now been discovered (HMSO 1965). Although the report emerged with reasonable speed, its recommendations took several years to be enacted. In the meantime, a very small problem had grown rapidly.

   An equally characteristic British response was the emergence of a number of voluntary organizations, in advance of statutory provision, designed to respond to the growing drug problem.

Early non-statutory drug services

The first non-statutory services were almost exclusively linked to Christian churches. Most began work with drug users in central London, providing befriending, some basic welfare work and counselling. In many ways they represented the classic missionary role of the Church, reaching out to those in distress. Thus Kenneth Leech at St Anne's, Soho, Barbara Ward, youth workers from the Salvation Army's Rink Club, Barbara Henry, Vic Ramsey at the Orange Street Mission, amongst others, began working in the streets, cafés and clubs of the West End, the theatre and entertainment centre of London, attempting to reach young drug users. Although each one was largely working alone, from their work a spate of new initiatives developed, emerging in the late 1960s into two distinctive groups. At one end, the first residential rehabilitation services were developed in Life for the World, the

New Life Foundation, and the Coke Hole Trust. At the other end, the first community drug services developed with the Soho Project and the Blenheim Project. The Community Drug Project stood out as a service which developed as a response to a local problem, inspired to a large extent by Griffith Edwards at the Addiction Research Unit.

By 1968, a new phase developed with services emerging from parent action, from concerned individuals and inspired by the experience of the United States. The Association for the Parents of Addicts, later renamed the Association for the Prevention of Addiction, was set up by Molly Craven in response to a family crisis. This spawned groups in many parts of the country, established a day centre in Covent Garden, and led to a number of services being established, many of which are still operating. In Hertfordshire, just to the north of London, Elizabeth Cory-Wright established the Hertfordshire Standing Conference on Drug Misuse, which despite a number of changes, still continues. In the second category, Terry Tanner and Ben Harrison set up ROMA (a residential rehabilitation project whose name derives from the acronym of their function of Rehabilitation Of Metropolitan Addicts) in response to the Advisory Committee on Drug Dependence report. Lord Longford established New Horizon, Eric Blakebrough opened Kaleidoscope, Peter Chapple set up CURE, the Institute for the Study of Drug Dependence (ISDD) was opened and the 'alternative society' was represented by the establishment of BIT and of Release to offer a legal and counselling service to those caught by the drug laws. (BIT was an organization providing information, emergency accommodation, legal advice, etc. to addicts. It was based in Westbourne Park, London.) In the final category came the 'concept-based' therapeutic communities. The leading ones were Alpha House in Portsmouth, Phoenix House in London, and slightly later Suffolk House in Iver Heath and the Ley Community in Oxford. Three of these were inspired by local consultant psychiatrists and were closely linked with a hospital-based service. Alpha House transferred to Hampshire Social Services Department and continued to be a statutory service provision well into the 1970s, although it moved out of St James's Hospital within a couple of years of opening.

The voluntary sector in the new drug services

By 1970, the pattern of voluntary and non-statutory services was established. They were almost the sole providers of drug-free residential rehabilitation, with many employing former drug users on the staff seeking to give a role model to residents. They provided the only accommodation specifically designed for drug users. And they offered day centres, outreach and detached work, advice and counselling services. The majority of these services employed paid staff, a few were exclusively provided by volunteers and many combined volunteer and paid staff.

A description of the history of voluntary organizations' work with drug users thus shows that they were at the heart of responses to drug problems in the 1960s. Whilst the haggling over the recommendations of the Brain Committee was continuing, they were opening services which have now become established approaches adopted over recent years by services provided by a range of non-statutory and statutory organizations.

What service was provided?

As importantly, the work undertaken by these services was a precursor to the services which are now commonly offered. In 1972, Ken Leech categorized the roles of the voluntary organizations into the following clusters: casualty caring, aftercare, education and agitators (Leech 1972). Those roles have barely changed, just the descriptors.

Casualty caring

Casualty caring included a wide range of activities, many now reintroduced under the rubric of 'harm reduction'. Detached and outreach work were common means of reaching drug users, as was the provision of peripatetic counselling and advisory services held in a variety of premises. The day centres provided kitchen and laundry facilities – I well remember the ingenuity which went into using up 1,000 cans of donated celery soup – found emergency accommodation, provided first aid and, perhaps more interestingly in light of modern developments, supplied needles and syringes whilst three out of the four had 'fixing rooms' where prescribed drugs could be injected in a relatively sterile and safe environment.

Aftercare

Aftercare was a broad concept. It included work with the probation service, prison visiting, preparation for release, and the development of accommodation and employment services. ROMA was designed to accommodate chaotic barbiturate and opiate users through a number of housing stages as stability developed leading on to independent flats, often for a family. AREA (Addict Rehabilitation Employment Agency), set up by Alee Reed, acted as an employment agency for drug users and those leaving rehabilitation. The range of residential services provided was in itself remarkable. As well as the concept-based therapeutic communities and the Christian houses, there were differing community models such as Par House, Cranstoun and Elizabeth House, and alternative communities such as the Patchwork Community, White Light, the Kingsway Community and Walnut Cottage. Perhaps it was inevitable that the alternative communities, so representative of an era, should not survive, but the loss of these agencies was also a loss of variety and opportunity which has never adequately been replaced.

Education

Education was represented in a variety of ways. A number of organizations provided information about drugs and addiction. Initially this was too close to propaganda and too far from accurate information. The emergence of ISDD, dedicated to non-partisan, accurate information and education, and of TACADE (the Teachers' Advisory Council on Alcohol and Drug Education) as a resource for school-based education had an increasing influence on the quality of the published material. In pre-video days, the production of films was also a common means of providing education. Project Icarus in Southampton was a major producer of education films, whilst James Ferman, later to be Secretary of the British Board of Film Censors, was responsible for the production of the first comprehensive set of drug education films. It is in the area of drug education that the greatest changes have occurred. In the 1960s and 1970s, education was almost exclusively concerned with limiting the likelihood of young people engaging in drug use. Now it has added limiting the likelihood of harm arising as a consequence of drug use.

Agitation

It was the role of voluntary organizations as agitators which Ken Leech feared was most likely to be lost as services became established. He had himself been one of the great agitators, almost achieving the same heartfelt cry from Kenneth Robinson, the then Minister of Health, as Thomas à Becket caused Henry II to make. His fears proved groundless. It was the voluntary organizations who found and exposed the corruption in the Metropolitan Drug Squad. They were at the heart of agitation for services in response to the needs of barbiturate users. They were advocates for their clients in court and with the treatment centres. Sometimes naive, they nevertheless were unquestionably on the side of their clients.

Change and consolidation during the 1970s

The 1970s was largely a period of consolidation and retrenchment. Few new services developed and a number closed. As public, political and press concern diminished and the impression was gained that drug use was declining, so the local action groups faded away and the army of volunteers disappeared. Many of the alternative communities closed or were forced to change to survive. The day centres also faced major challenges. As treatment centres changed to prescribing oral drugs, the day centre clients who continued to inject were using illicit drugs and barbiturates. Staff were forced increasingly into policing the centres, managing overdoses and administering first aid. The fixing rooms were no longer viable when those who most needed them had to be denied because their drug use was illicit and overdose a common consequence. By 1975, all the fixing rooms had closed and needles and syringes were no longer supplied. It was ironic that the agitation for a crisis service for barbiturate users which began at the start of the 1970s did not result in a service, City Roads (Crisis Intervention), until the barbiturate problem was rapidly declining and the new problems of the 1980s beginning to emerge. For the residential services it was also a time of change. The concept-based therapeutic communities threw off the shackles of their American genesis and began to develop a British identity, with some of the more extreme aspects of the programme, such as the shaving of heads and the wearing of placards announcing the residents' faults, being abandoned. ROMA closed, transferred ownership and reopened as a compact version of its original vision. By 1981, the total number of specialist drug services operated by non-statutory organizations was forty, with about the same number of specialist hospital services.[1]

The formation of SCODA

In 1971, the non-statutory organizations had agreed the need for improved co-ordination and co-operation and as a result established SCODA, the Standing Conference on Drug Abuse, which acted as an umbrella organization for voluntary sector projects, and which employed its first staff in 1972. By 1978, its members were reporting an increasing number of young heroin users approaching them seeking help. Once more the role as agitators came to the fore as efforts were made to achieve a commitment of resources so that drug services could be expanded to meet a growing need. The response was not dissimilar to that in the 1960s. First denial, then a call for more information and finally, in 1982, publication of 'Treatment and Rehabilitation' (Advisory Council on the Misuse of Drugs, 1982) with the announcement of additional central funding.

Rapid growth during the 1980s

The 1980s saw non-statutory drug services develop rapidly, not only in the number and variety of services they offered, but also as influencers of policy. They produced their own critique of the *Treatment and rehabilitation* report and a framework for the development of services (SCODA 1983). They challenged the draft circular on the Central Funding Initiative and submitted an alternative, which was adopted by the Department of Health almost unchanged. They prepared the guidance for monitoring services funded under the initiative. They prepared the first advice note on AIDS and drug use and developed guidance for services. They developed quality standards for service provision which have become a benchmark against which services can be measured. They campaigned for the exclusion of drug addiction as a sole basis for compulsory admission to a psychiatric hospital and for the inclusion of residential drug services within the terms of the Residential Homes Act.

The Central Funding Initiative, undertaken by the Department of Health, made dedicated funds available which provided the basis for the rapid growth of drug services throughout England. There were separate initiatives undertaken by the Welsh Office and the Scottish Office. The two main strands of service provision were community-based services and residential services. The former were subdivided between statutory provision, commonly referred to as Community Drug Teams, and non-statutory provision of advice, counselling and information services. The residential services continued to be the exclusive provision of non-statutory organizations, with an increasing number of fee-paying services being established.

So what promotes voluntary sector growth?

There were a number of similarities to the development of drug services in the 1960s and early 1970s, although the differences may be more significant. The services of the 1960s and 1970s were primarily centred on London, concerned with a small but significant number of people with acute drug problems. Their clients had multiple problems with many who had migrated to London,[2] had been in care, were homeless and unemployed. By the 1980s, drug problems were reported throughout the country and services were opened to respond to this development. Moreover, the new drug users were predominantly smoking heroin rather than injecting, were still living at home or in their home area and were relatively young.[3] The older services, developed to work with a very different pattern of drug use, had difficulty in responding to this change.

A number of new services emerged as a result of community and parent action. This often led to conflict with established services, both statutory and non-statutory. They were, in many ways, replicating the development process of the 1960 services which challenged the perceived complacency and inaction of the 'authorities'. There were two strands to parent action. One was concerned with direct service provision, leading to services such as CADA (Committee Against Drug Abuse, who set up a drop-in centre in south London) and Drugline in south London, Drugline in Birmingham, and the Place in Glasgow. The other was concerned with self-help and mutual support with the establishment of Families Anonymous and ADFAM and a range of local groups. Even here, there were echoes of the 1960s and the work of the APA (Association for the Prevention of Addiction).

In the mid-1980s, the increased awareness of HIV infection and its possible consequences led to a further flurry of pioneering activity. Innovations in providing health information to drug users, such as *Smack in the Eye* produced by the Lifeline Project in Manchester, and *Drug Alert*, broadcast by BBC Radio One[4] based on ideas developed by SCODA, represented a move away from prevention as an absolute – don't start, and if you have, stop – to an understanding of prevention in personal and public health terms where avoiding or reducing harm was important and relevant to drug and non-drug users. There were also reinventions of past practice with the development of needle and syringe exchange schemes and the reintroduction of outreach and detached work. The difference between the 1960s/1970s and the 1980s/1990s was that in the former, the pioneers were innocents who tried new approaches with little experience to go on, with no clear outcome identified as the goal and with no evaluation of the approaches they tried. In the latter, the majority were less often pioneers and more often drug worker professionals who were cautious of taking too many risks but were willing to push the boundaries of accepted practice to the limits without over-stretching the mark. This caution was reinforced because of the threats to funding and to services observed when drug services were regarded as having gone too far, for instance by publishing leaflets which did not outrightly condemn drugs or particular drugs, or in promoting safer injecting where a drug user was unwilling to stop injecting altogether.

The drive towards professionalization

This caution perhaps reflected some of the changes which had occurred and continued to occur in the 1990s. Specialist drug services now comprise professional groups seeking to be recognized as such. The demand for formal qualifications as a basis for being employed in drug services is increasing, as is the demand for post-qualification training which will lead to a further qualification in addiction counselling, or addictions or some similar title. Nevertheless, the drugs field is still staffed by a workforce with low levels of relevant training (Boys *et al.*, 1997). The internal pressure for status has been matched by the external pressure arising from changes in the way services are funded and the controls which will be put on them.

New legislation affecting health, social and probation services, changes in charity law and in the regulations of other statutory funding sources is in danger of enforcing a new orthodoxy. Professional standards of management, detailed case recording and assessment procedures, quality assurance, performance measurement, service audit, all these are beginning to appear within contracts for service as they replace grants as the main source of funding for non-statutory services. Whilst there can be no doubt that drug users, like any other service user or customer, have the right to high quality services, there is the danger that the variety of services will be lost and that a smaller number of services will become excellent for the few who wish to use them. Pioneering will revert to the under-resourced outsiders, the agitators, as the distinction between statutory and non-statutory services continues to blur.

However, this gloomy picture may be challenged by another glance at the 1960s and early 1970s. Non-statutory services have been at the forefront of developments for more than thirty years and they have had the opportunity to develop that role within the new legislation. Community care and health-care planning requires that customers of services are consulted in the development of plans and that services respond to the needs of the community. Already there are developing support and action groups of drug users to some extent modelled on the Junkiebond in the Netherlands. The role of the agitator, or in today's language, advocate, for drug users, their right to services and to services which are relevant to their needs has re-emerged as a key function.

Conclusion

There will inevitably be conflicts between the different possible objectives of public policy in responding to drug problems. The demand for increased international action, for improved enforcement and for deterrence will at times be in conflict with public health, social and health-care needs. There will be conflict with those who wish to establish orthodoxy and the blandness of a uniform approach. For non-statutory services, their future mission must be to be agitators for services based on, and supported by, an assessment of the needs of their customers.

There is still a need for pioneers. The roles identified by Kenneth Leech thirty years ago remain as valid now as then. The difference is that those roles can be pressed as insiders where drug users have rights within the broad citizens' charter and within the framework of service planning and where non-statutory services can be partners as agitators and advocates for service.

Notes

1 Although many more hospitals were listed as 'known to be providing some facilities for the treatment of drug addiction', the majority only offered general psychiatric out-patient appointments or in-patient detoxification in a general psychiatric ward. Some 45 hospitals had specialist treatment units.
2 For instance, in 1972 New Horizon reported that some 50 per cent of their clients were from Scotland, primarily from the west coast. Similar experiences reported from other London services resulted in the Scots Group being established to develop links with organizations in Scotland and to seek means to reduce this migration.

3 By 1983, almost 50 per cent of new addict notifications were under 25 years of age although the percentage of addicts under 25 years recorded as receiving notifiable drugs in treatment at the end of the year remained stable at about 19 per cent.
4 Radio One is the popular music channel in the UK with a weekly audience reach of about 17 million people, the vast majority under 30 years of age.

References

Advisory Committee on Drug Dependence (1969). *The rehabilitation of drug addicts*. HMSO, London.

Advisory Council on the Misuse of Drugs (1982). *Treatment and rehabilitation*. HMSO, London.

Boys, A., Strang, J. and Homan, C. (1997). Have drug workers in England received appropriate training?: 1995 baseline data from a national survey. *Drugs: Education, Prevention and Policy*, 4: 297–304.

Drug addiction. Report of the Interdepartmental Committee (1961). HMSO, London.

Drug addiction. The Second Report of the Interdepartmental Committee (1965). HMSO, London.

Leech, K. (1972). The role of the voluntary agencies. *British Journal of Addiction*, 67: 131–6.

SCODA (1983). Response of SCODA to the Report of the Advisory Council on the Misuse of Drugs: Treatment and Rehabilitation. SCODA, London.

Chapter 16

AIDS and drug misuse in the UK

Achievements, failings and new harm reduction opportunities

John Strang

(This chapter draws substantially on material originally published in journal form as: Strang, J. (1998) AIDS and drug misuse – 10 years on: achievements, failings and new harm reduction opportunities. *Drugs, Education, Policy and Prevention*, 5: 293–304.)

The threat of AIDS forced a major re-appraisal of policy and practice in the UK (Advisory Council on the Misuse of Drugs (ACMD), 1988; Strang and Stimson, 1990) which was the marker of a significant shift in the evolving 'British System' (Strang, 1989; Strang and Gossop, 1994). This new perspective involved a broader consideration of the public health issues, and led to changes in existing treatment services as well as new HIV-specific services. However, there are also areas of 'intervention inertia' in which policy makers and practitioners have failed to implement essential change, as well as further areas of potential harm reduction yield which have not yet been seriously explored (Strang, 1992). More than a decade later, it is appropriate to take stock of the situation and to describe some of the successes, reflect on the failures, and speculate on possible new areas of development in the harm reduction field.

In this chapter, four particular areas are considered. First, what was new about the health risk facing the broader population of drug injectors – and how did this lead to the public health approach that was adopted to dealing with the problems of HIV amongst injecting drug misusers? Second, an examination is required as to how concerns about HIV transmission have brought a new focus to the work of existing treatment services, as well as being the birthright of the new services established in the wake of HIV awareness. Third, the spotlight should be shone on those areas in which we have failed to respond adequately, and a consideration should be made of the reasons underlying these disappointing failures of policy and practice. Fourth, an exploration is necessary in order to chart some of the new areas in which it may be possible for new harm reduction opportunities to be developed.

Implications from considering a broader target population

First, it is necessary to note the very different and novel context of the harm reduction debate in the late 1980s. The intense harm reduction debate in the drugs field had been largely prompted by the recognition that HIV was being transmitted from one injecting drug misuser to another (and thence to their sexual partners and further into the broader community) through the sharing of injecting equipment.

In the UK, the government's Advisory Council on the Misuse of Drugs produced its influential report on AIDS and Drug Misuse in 1988, in which it reported on its crucial first conclusion that: 'HIV is a greater threat to public and individual health than drug misuse', and that the first goal of work with drug misusers must therefore be to prevent them from acquiring or transmitting the virus. As they pointed out, in some cases this will be achieved through abstinence, whilst for others, abstinence will not be achievable for the time being and efforts will need to focus on risk reduction (ACMD, 1988, 1989).

For many, one of the important component parts of the harm reduction debate was the stepping aside from any moral judgements. The advocate of harm reduction was neither for nor against personal freedoms; neither for nor against changes in the legal status of drug use; neither for nor against changes in treatment provision – except insofar as they could be shown to have a direct relationship to the amounts of harm which resulted for an individual and for society (Strang, 1992). Hence drug policy was seen as quite properly fitting alongside other areas of public policy and public health strategy, where the public health physician recognized that, whilst aware that moral positions may be taken with regard to the behaviour, their task was to concentrate on achieving reductions in the harms identified (Heather et al., 1993).

An important early observation in the review prompted by HIV concerned the large numbers of injecting drug users who were believed to exist in the wider population but who were not in treatment (ACMD, 1988). Insofar as they might acquire or transmit HIV infection, they were a vital target population for public health planning. However, in considering those not in treatment, it was insufficient merely to look at ways of increasing treatment capacity so as to be able to recruit them into treatment. For some of these non-treatment drug injectors, there may either be no suitable treatment with which to attract them, or it may simply be that they had no perception of any problem with their drug use and did not wish to receive treatment. For the drug injector who did not see his or her drug misuse as a problem, the concept of treatment would have seemed absurd. Yet such non-treatment-seeking injectors were nevertheless the target of an essential part of the public policy formation even if they did not wish to be involved in individual treatment.

Policy-makers also needed to think beyond just the current injector. Injecting drug misusers were the obvious first target group for the public health planning: however, it was necessary to extend the consideration to those whose drug use, whilst not actually currently involving injecting, involved a drug which was often injected (and hence were at major risk of becoming tomorrow's injectors) – See Figure 16.1.

Thus, when considering heroin users, interest turned to the large numbers of new young heroin users who were taking their heroin by 'chasing the dragon' (Gossop *et al.*, 1988; Strang *et al.*, 1992a; Griffiths *et al.*, 1994a) – a phenomenon which swept across many cities in the UK during the 1980s. These heroin chasers were likely to include many of tomorrow's injectors, as the drug transitions studies in London were finding a substantial progression on to injecting by these former non-injecting heroin users (Griffiths *et al.*, 1994b; Strang *et al.*, 1997a).

The impact on clinical practice of a broader public health approach

What were the practical implications of considering this broader target population – the population of drug misusers 'out there' and not just only those in treatment? First, there was the need to distribute public information on the dangers of needle sharing (and the potential for sexual transmission), through the ordinary channels of posters and press and television advertising.

From 1985 onwards, information about the importance of HIV risk became progressively more widespread, and, from 1987 onwards, posters were widely displayed which were aimed specifically at the hidden populations of injecting drug misusers.

Additionally, information on cleaning contaminated needles and syringes in emergencies was provided – not only by local drug agencies but also by the Department of Health, as shown in Figure 16.2, a reproduction from the Department of Health 1991 Guidelines (DoH, 1991). This represents an excellent example of the acceptance of the imperfect – that although one might wish the injecting drug misuser always to use clean needles and syringe, it must nevertheless be recognized that there will be occasions when the drug injector may, against the guidance, use a previously-used needle and syringe. Although the main message would be one of complete hygiene around the technique, it is nevertheless vital to provide information on how to clean needles and syringes in an emergency.

From 1987 onwards, a network of needle and syringe exchange schemes was established across the UK (Stimson *et al.*, 1988, 1990), often linked with outreach workers (ACMD, 1993; Rhodes, 1993), and built on a public health planning approach. They were not linked to entry into treatment, but addressed the injecting behaviour of the wider drug-injecting population. In addition, needles and syringes have become increasingly available for sale

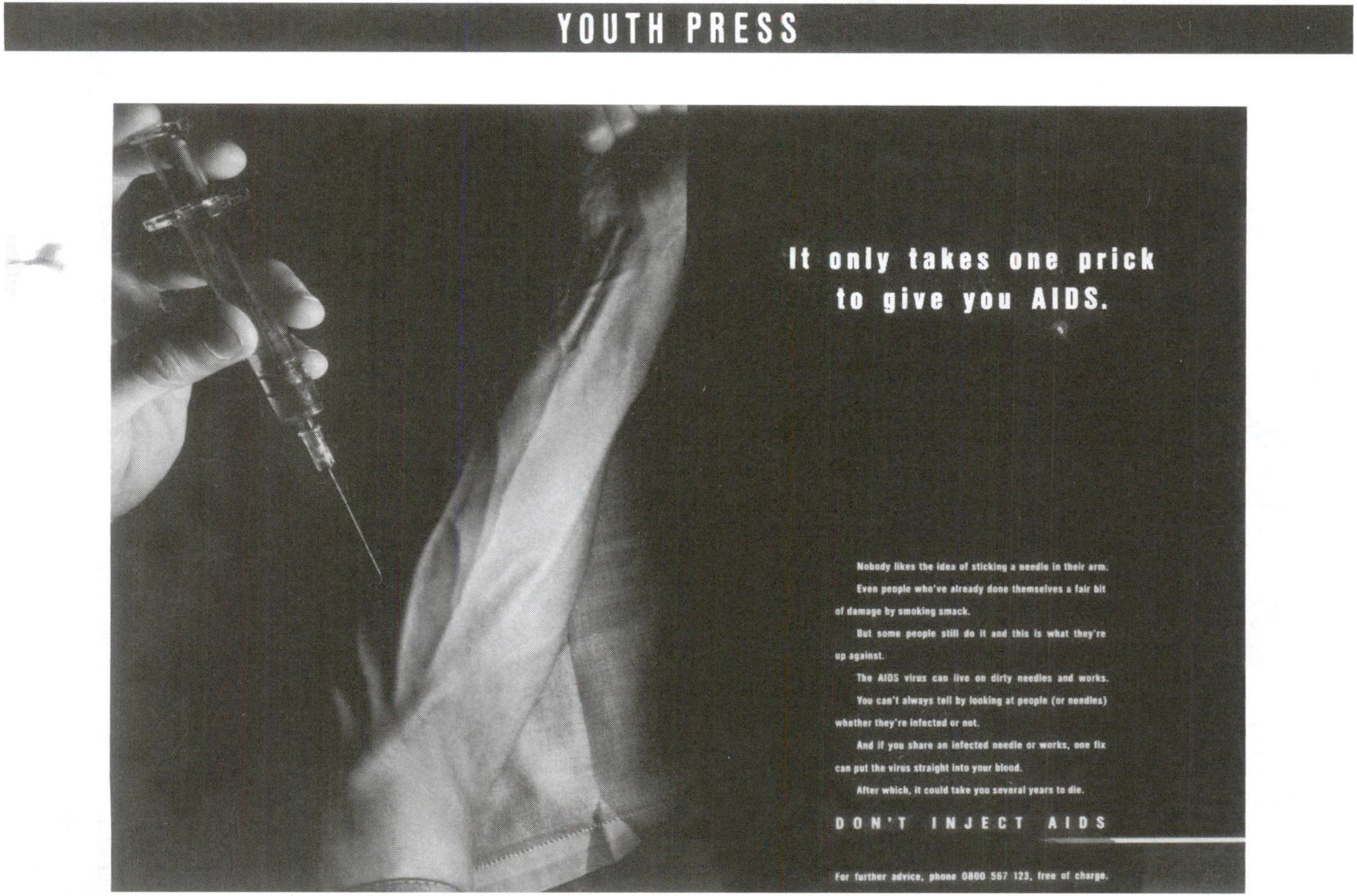

Figure 16.1 It only takes one prick to give you AIDS
Source: Department of Health.

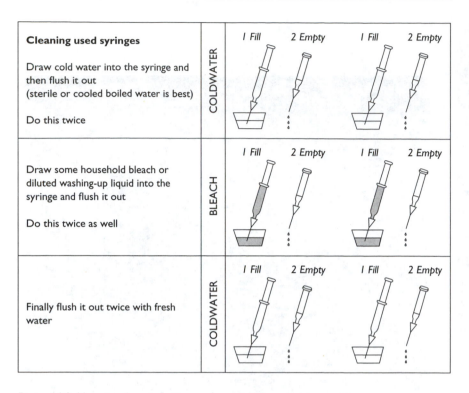

Cleaning used syringes Draw cold water into the syringe and then flush it out (sterile or cooled boiled water is best) Do this twice	COLDWATER	*1 Fill*	*2 Empty*	*1 Fill*	*2 Empty*
Draw some household bleach or diluted washing-up liquid into the syringe and flush it out Do this twice as well	BLEACH	*1 Fill*	*2 Empty*	*1 Fill*	*2 Empty*
Finally flush it out twice with fresh water	COLDWATER	*1 Fill*	*2 Empty*	*1 Fill*	*2 Empty*

Figure 16.2 How to clean injecting equipment if it must be reused
Source: Adapted from a 'Mainliners' leaflet, Department of Health Guidelines (1991).

from community pharmacies (Sheridan *et al.*, 1996, 2000) and at least as many needles and syringes were being used which were from this source as were from the dedicated needle and syringe exchange schemes. Over the last decade, community pharmacies have also become increasingly involved in needle and syringe exchange, and many are willing to provide free 'sharps boxes' for the injecting drug user to take away (Sheridan *et al.*, 1997) and this has included the development of explicit pharmacy-based needle and syringe exchange schemes (Sheridan *et al.*, 2000).

Perhaps the most important impact of HIV on existing treatments was the greater clarity of purpose around changing injecting and sharing behaviour (Strang, 1988). Through the 1980s, therapeutic work with drug users had moved increasingly to being assistance through a process of change in which the drug users had reached a point of contemplation about their drug use, aware of the costs as well as the advantages which they saw as associated with their drug use – work very different from the maintenance prescribing of the early 1970s (Stimson and Oppenheimer, 1982; Strang, 1984; Stimson, 1987). In addition to helping the drug misuser conduct this personal cost–benefit analysis, drug agencies were also wishing to be more involved in helping the drug misuser to implement some action (such as becoming drug-free) and in maintaining this new state (e.g. remaining drug-free). However, with the attention to the benefits of intermediate goals (i.e. goals which were short of abstinence) (ACMD, 1988), the new view of treatment changed to one in which it might be seen as working through a cascade of processes of change (Strang, 1990). Thus, to illustrate, the first process of change might be to assist the drug user to disengage from his/her criminal behaviour, whilst the second cascade might be to assist him/her in ceasing all sharing of injecting equipment, with the third process of change being to move away from injecting. However, whilst there has been great enthusiasm for this attention to intermediate goals, it must also be acknowledged that great difficulties have been encountered with this approach with the patient failing to make progress through such a cascade. Whilst attractive, and in some ways elegant, the system only works efficiently if there is movement through the cascade, and hence concern has been expressed (ACMD, 1993; Strang, 1994) about naive interpretations of the process of change.

Gradually, the UK is moving towards greater reliance on evidence from international research in the addictions field (e.g. Department of Health Task Force, 1996). There is now a much better understanding of the importance of retaining the patient in treatment, with treatment retention being related to more durable and greater healthy behaviour change. This evidence base has been most impressive with structured oral methadone maintenance programmes (e.g. Farrell et al., 1994; Ward et al., 1999), with the greatest benefits being seen with high-dose oral methadone maintenance, delivered in a treatment programme which combines the broader elements of a therapeutic programme with the specific pharmacotherapeutic approach.

A watchful eye needs to be kept on the new pharmacotherapies which are becoming available in the addictions field internationally. Methadone is now more than half a century old as a drug, and has been widely used in the addictions field for over 30 years. One of the new drugs of potential interest is buprenorphine, the mixed agonist–antagonist drug (Strain et al., 1994), although better information is required about the possibility of combining this drug with naloxone in view of the problems in the UK with intravenous use of buprenorphine (Sakol et al., 1989).

Areas of failure and unjustified inertia

It is also possible to identify areas in which we seem to have failed. Whilst the low extent to which HIV has spread amongst our drug-using populations has prompted modest self-congratulation (Stimson, 1995, 1996), the wide prevalence of hepatitis C infection is a surprising and disturbing cause for concern (Coutinho, 1998). Over what is probably a similar period, hepatitis C infection has become widespread amongst injecting drug misusers. To illustrate, a recent study in south London found that 70 per cent of addicts in treatment were already positive for hepatitis C (Best *et al.*, 1999). Furthermore, this includes drug users whose history of injecting is relatively recent (Noble *et al.*, 2000), and hence would seem to indicate a continued level of risk behaviour – at least sufficient to transmit the hepatitis C virus. More attention certainly needs to be paid to the dynamics of hepatitis C in this population, as the hepatitis viruses will be leading to enormous harm in this population over the years ahead (see Chapter 17, this volume).

We must also be vigilant about the extent to which transitions (Strang *et al.*, 1992b) may occur from smoking to injecting. During the 1980s and 1990s, in many cities in the UK, 'chasing the dragon' became the main route for new initiation into heroin use (Burr, 1987; Gossop *et al.*, 1988; Parker *et al.*, 1987, 1988; Pearson, 1987; Pearson *et al.*, 1986). With rapidly growing numbers of young people involved in 'chasing the dragon', HIV prevention strategy in the UK needs to maintain a careful watch on the proportions of these heroin chasers who subsequently move on to injecting. At present the picture remains unclear, and certainly needs careful scrutiny and further study.

But perhaps the greatest wasted opportunity for intervention is in our prisons in the UK. The prison system had more contact with injecting drug misusers than any other agency (ACMD, 1996; Farrell and Strang, 1991; Harding, 1990). Sadly, perhaps because prisons are seen as concerned almost exclusively with control and punishment, we have been slow and inefficient at harnessing the therapeutic opportunities. Although not sought voluntarily, the period of imprisonment offers an excellent opportunity for health education and for orientation about alternatives to drug-using lifestyles, as well as offering an excellent opportunity for routine health checks and hepatitis B immunization, for example. And yet, in most prisons in the UK, a set of circumstances has long prevailed in which even the most basic provision of detoxification has usually not been available. Slowly the prison system is becoming more responsible with regard to utilizing these health opportunities, but, 15 years after the Advisory Council on the Misuse of Drugs first drew attention to the important opportunity in prisons, the progress has still been insufficient, and many of the changes called for (ACMD, 1988, 1989, 1993, 1996) are still not yet widely available outside a limited number of demonstration projects.

It must also be remembered that the treatment itself may bring harm. One obvious area of possible harm is with diversion of prescribed supplies of drugs on to the black market. In the UK there still exists an extraordinarily unregulated system for prescribing and dispensing. Through the 1990s there was a four-fold increase in the number of opiate addicts receiving treatment with methadone (Strang *et al.*, 1996a). Yet, despite such a major expansion of this type of treatment, only scant attention is paid to control and supervision. Virtually all prescriptions for methadone are on a take-home basis, with a third of all methadone prescriptions being for take-home instalments of at least a week's supply (Strang *et al.*, 1996a; Strang and Sheridan, 2003) – hence the scope for diversion is enormous, and, as a consequence, there exists a major problem of a black market in these prescribed supplies of methadone, leading to worries about their contribution to overdose deaths amongst drug misusers (Cairns *et al.*, 1996; McCarthy, 1997). Additionally, there must be legitimate anxiety and concern that the treatment itself may be prolonging the injecting career or at least the opiate career of the drug misuser – that instead of facilitating flow through a process of change, the provision of a prescribed supply of the drug may sometimes act as an obstructor to change (Strang, 1990, 1994; Strang *et al.*, 1998). Despite the encouraging evidence that oral methadone maintenance helps the opiate addict move away from injecting, no such benefit is likely to occur with injectable maintenance prescribing, which, if anything, may be reinforcing the behavioural pattern of injecting (Battersby *et al.*, 1992). Hence there should be even more determination that there must be demonstrable evidence of healthy behaviour change if we are considering prescribing injectable drugs.

Public intrigue with some particular aspects of the drug policy debate can perhaps distract attention onto issues which may be of great media fascination but are actually of less true importance. Much of the media fascination with heroin-prescribing in the UK could perhaps be seen as in this category, where the widespread expansion of oral methadone maintenance programmes in the UK was held back for many years because so much passion was being expended on debates around whether or not the extremely small amount of heroin-prescribing should be increased or decreased. Similarly, in the UK development of needle and syringe exchange schemes, a disproportionate amount of time and energy has been spent in debating whether or not sterile water ampoules and sterile swabs should be provided for injecting drug misusers – rather than concentrating on increasing further the availability of equipment and the thoroughness of the collection of used needles and syringes.

New territories not yet adequately explored

Finally, is it possible to identify new territories in which harm reduction strategies could valuably be employed? One of the great legacies of the drugs/HIV debate of the last decade has been the appropriate re-focusing of policy and practice objectives to reductions of individual and public harms, and this new perspective can valuably be applied beyond consideration of HIV.

From the point of view of community benefit, the impressive evidence about reduced criminal activities of opiate addicts recruited into methadone maintenance programmes (Gossop *et al.*, 1996a; Hubbard *et al.*, 1989; Simpson *et al.*, 1986; Strang *et al.*, 1997b) stands as an example of reducing the overall harm to society. This is a valuable new way of viewing public policy formation, in which the harm in society is gauged under different circumstances and then mechanisms found which reduce the extent of this harm. But more explicitly health-focused new possible harm reduction strategies can also be identified.

The opportunity to immunize against hepatitis B stands as an excellent opportunity (Department of Health Task Force, 1996; Polkinghorne *et al.*, 1997) which is currently being missed in most drug treatment services in the UK (Farrell *et al.*, 1990; Mangtani *et al.*, 1995, 1996; Winstock *et al.*, 2000), and elsewhere in the world. In UK studies, about half of injecting drug misusers already have markers indicating past infection with hepatitis B (Gossop *et al.*, 1994) whilst, for the other half, they have not yet been infected – although the proportion infected steadily increases with increasing duration of injecting career (Noble *et al.*, 2000). Hence, these hepatitis B negative injecting drug misusers constitute a population in which huge benefit could be conferred by the provision of hepatitis B immunization, which would not only benefit the individual drug misusers themselves but also their future injecting and sexual partners. Sadly, the continuing failure of drug agencies to incorporate hepatitis B immunization into their routine practice (Farrell *et al.*, 1990; Mangtani *et al.*, 1996; Winstock *et al.*, 2000) is largely as a result of resistance on the part of drug workers, their agency managers and funders to address an explicitly medical problem and to take seriously the long-term physical well-being of their clients.

For the next possible harm reduction territory, the exciting work which has been undertaken in the alcohol (Chick *et al.*, 1985; Wallace *et al.*, 1988) and smoking fields (Kottke *et al.*, 1988; Russell *et al.*, 1979) with regard to brief interventions should be examined. A wide range of services now have passing contact with an extended population of injecting drug misusers – for example, the huge number of brief contacts with injecting drug misusers whilst they purchase needles and syringes from community pharmacies or obtain free supplies from needle and syringe exchange schemes. There is obviously enormous opportunity for the delivery of brief interventions, if we were able to develop these and demonstrate that benefit could be conferred in this manner. This is one of the possible new areas of harm reduction work which should be taken more seriously henceforth.

As a final example of a possible new territory for harm reduction, prevention of the morbidity and mortality which result from opiate overdoses warrants consideration. In both the UK and Australian studies of the personal overdose experiences of treatment and community samples of injecting drug misusers (Darke *et al.*, 1995a, 1995b; Gossop *et al.*; 1996b; Powis *et al.*, 1999), between a third and half have personally experienced an overdose. Perhaps even more startling is that about a fifth had actually been present at a fatal overdose (Strang *et al.*, 1999). Virtually all of these overdoses involved use of heroin – either alone or in conjunction with other drugs. Of particular concern was the lack of knowledge about proper management of such overdoses. Sometimes other drugs were additionally injected in an attempt to resuscitate the fellow drug misuser, and extensive delays occurred before an ambulance was called (Best *et al.*, 2002). Basic provision of cardiopulmonary resuscitation was rare. Perhaps serious consideration should be given to the possibility of teaching for drug misusers in treatment about basic cardiopulmonary resuscitation, and possibly also to the provision of emergency supplies of naloxone (the injectable rapid-acting opiate antagonist) which they might administer to a fellow drug misuser who has overdosed (Strang *et al.*, 1996a). By such methods, it is probable that the vast majority of the witnessed overdose fatalities could have been avoided (Strang *et al.*, 1999; Dettmer *et al.*, 2002). It is surprising that such approaches have not been employed, or at least debated previously; might it be that they constitute too great an affront to public and professional perceptions of the level of self-efficacy of drug misusers?

Conclusion

During the late 1980s, there was, within the UK, a successful reorientation of drug policy, with a serious embracing of the public health imperative of stemming the transmission of HIV (ACMD, 1988, 1989; Strang and Stimson, 1990). The policies and practices adopted were mostly not new, but were drawn from pre-existing principles of public health – but they needed to be brought to the fore in terms of new policy formation.

This created a climate in which it was possible to establish new types of service, such as the network of needle and syringe exchange schemes (Stimson *et al.*, 1988, 1990) and also more widely available methadone treatment (Farrell *et al.*, 1994; Strang *et al.*, 1996b; Strang and Sheridan 2003).

Despite these encouraging observations, there are still resistant 'black spots' in which policy and practice fail to deal adequately with the challenge of HIV risk reduction, and similarly the risks of infection with other viruses such as hepatitis B and hepatitis C (Department of Health Task Force, 1996). Our continued failure to use health opportunities in prisons stands as one of the resistant black spots (ACMD, 1993, 1996; Harding, 1990).

Opportunities exist for taking forward recent work or harm reduction, identifying new areas of possible intervention and new forms of existing harm which can be reduced by these approaches. Policy makers and practitioners will need to stand apart from the moral debate and concentrate on promoting strategies for the acquisition of health gains at the individual and public health levels. Knowledge, discipline and integrity will be required in equal measure to follow through in these new exciting areas.

References

Advisory Council on the Misuse of Drugs (1988). AIDS and Drugs Misuse (Part 1) Report. London: HMSO.

Advisory Council on the Misuse of Drugs (1989). AIDS and Drug Misuse (Part 2) Report. London: HMSO.

Advisory Council on the Misuse of Drugs (1993). AIDS and Drugs Misuse: Update report. London: HMSO.

Advisory Council on the Misuse of Drugs (1996). Drug Misusers and the Prison system – an integrated approach. Report of the Criminal Justice Working Group, Part 3. London: HMSO.

Battersby, M., Strang, J., Farrell, M., Gossop, M. and Robson, P. (1992). 'Horsetrading': prescribing injectable opiates to opiate addicts – a descriptive study. *Drug and Alcohol Review*, 11, pp. 35–42.

Best, D., Noble, A., Finch, E., Gossop, M., Sidwell, C. and Strang, J. (1999). Accuracy of perceptions of hepatitis B and C status: cross sectional investigation of opiate addicts in treatment. *British Medical Journal*, 319, pp. 290–91.

Burr, A. (1987). Chasing the dragon: heroin misuse, delinquency and crime in the context of South London culture. *British Journal of Criminology*, 27, pp. 333–57.

Cairns, A., Roberts, I. and Benbow, E. (1996). Characteristics of fatal methadone overdoses in Manchester, 1985–1994. *British Medical Journal*, 313, pp. 264–65.

Chick, J., Lloyd, G. and Crombie, E. (1985). Counselling problem drinkers in medical wards: a controlled study. *British Medical Journal*, 290, pp. 965–67.

Coutinho, R. A. (1998). HIV and hepatitis C among injecting drug users: success in preventing HIV has not been mirrored for hepatitis C. *British Medical Journal*, 317, pp. 424–25.

Darke, S., Ross, J. and Hall, W. (1995a). Overdose among heroin users in Sydney, Australia – 1. Prevalence and correlates of non-fatal overdose. *Addiction*, 91, pp. 405–11.

Darke, S., Ross, J. and Hall, W. (1995b). Overdose among heroin users in Sydney, Australia – 2. Responses to overdose. *Addiction*, 91, pp. 413–17.

Department of Health (1991). Drug Misuse and Dependence: guidelines on clinical management. London: HMSO.

Department of Health Task Force (1996). The Task Force to Review Services for Drug Misusers: report of an independent review of drug treatment services in England. London: HMSO.

Dettmer, K., Saunders, W. and Strang, J. (2001). Take home naloxone and the prevention of deaths from opiate overdose: two pilot schemes. *British Medical Journal*, 322, pp. 895–96.

Farrell, M. and Strang, J. (1991). Drugs and HIV in prisons: the hole in the net. *British Medical Journal*, 302, pp. 1477–78.

Farrell, M., Battersby, M. and Strang, J. (1990). Screening for hepatitis B and vaccination of injecting drug users in NHS drug treatment services. *British Journal of Addiction*, 85, pp. 1657–59.

Farrell, M., Ward, J., Des Jarlais, D. C., Gossop, M., Stimson, G., Hall, W., Matttck, R. and Strang, J. (1994). Methadone maintenance programmes: review of new data with special reference to impact on HIV transmission. *British Medical Journal*, 309, pp. 997–1001.

Gossop, M., Griffiths, P. and Strang, J. (1988). 'Chasing the dragon': a comparison of heroin chasers and injectors seen by a London community drug team. *British Journal of Addiction*, 83, pp. 1159–62.

Gossop, M., Marsden, J., Edwards, C., Wilson, A., Seagar, G., Stewart, D. and Lehmann, P. (1996a). NTORS: The National Treatment Outcome Research Study – a report to the Department of Health. London: HMSO (reported in Department of Health Task Force Report).

Gossop, M., Griffiths, P., Powis, B., Williamson, S. and Strang, J. (1996b). Frequency of non-fatal heroin overdose: survey of heroin users recruited in non-clinical settings. *British Medical Journal*, 313, p. 402.

Gossop, M., Powis, B., Griffiths, P. and Strang, J. (1994). Interaction of multiple risks for HIV and hepatitis B infection amongst heroin users. *Drug and Alcohol Review*, 13, pp. 293–300.

Griffiths, P., Gossop, M. and Strang, J. (1994a). Chasing the dragon: the development of heroin smoking in the United Kingdom. In J. Strang and M. Gossop (eds), *Heroin Addiction and Drug Policy: 'The British System'* (pp. 121–33). Oxford: Oxford University Press.

Griffiths. P., Gossop, M., Powis, B. and Strang, J. (1994b). Transitions in patterns of heroin administration: a study of heroin chasers and heroin injectors. *Addiction*, 89, pp. 301–9.

Harding, T. (1990). HIV infection and AIDS in the prison environment: a test case for the respect of human rights. In J. Strang and G. V. Stimson (eds), *AIDS and Drug Misuse: the challenge for policy and practice in the 1990s* (pp. 197–209). London: Routledge.

Heather, N., Wodak, A. and O'Hare, P. (1993). *Harm Reduction: from faith to science*. London: Whurr Publishers.

Hubbard, R. L., Marsden, M. E., Rachal, J. V., Harwood, H. J., Cavanagh, E. R. and Ginzburg, H. M. (1989). *Drug Abuse Treatment: a national study of effectiveness*. Carolina, USA: University of North Carolina Press.

Kottke, T. E., Battista, R. N., De Friese, G. H. and Brekkem, L. (1988). Attributes of successful smoking cessation interventions in medical practice: a meta analysis of 39 controlled trials. *Journal of the American Medical Association*, 259, pp. 2883–89.

Mangtani, P., Hall, A. and Normand, C. E. (1995). Hepatitis B vaccination: the cost effectiveness of alternative strategies in England and Wales. *Journal of Epidemiology and Community Health*, 49, pp. 238–44.

Mangtani, P., Kovats, S. and Hall, A. (1996). Hepatitis B vaccination policy in drug treatment services (letter). *British Medical Journal*, 311, p. 1500.

McCarthy, J. H. (1997). More people die from methadone misuse than heroin misuse. *British Medical Journal*, 315, p. 603.

Noble, A., Best, D., Finch, E., Gossop, M., Sidwell, C. and Strang, J. (2000). Injecting risk behaviour and year of first infection as predictors of hepatitis B and C status among methadone maintenance patients in south London. *Journal of Substance Use*, 5: 131–35.

Parker, H., Bakx, K. and Newcombe, R. (1988). *Living with Heroin*. Milton Keynes: Open University Press.

Parker, H., Newcombe, R. and Bakx, K. (1987). The new heroin users: prevalence and characteristics in the Wirral, Merseyside. *British Journal of Addiction*, 82, pp. 147–58.

Pearson, G. (1987). *The New Heroin Users*. Oxford: Blackwell.

Pearson, G., Gilman, M. and McIver, S. (1986). Heroin use in the North of England. *Health Education Journal*, 45, pp. 186–89.

Polkinghorne, J., Strang, J. and Farrell, M. (1997). Mistake in report: hepatitis B vaccination for drug misusers is recommended. *British Medical Journal*, 315, p. 61.

Powis, B., Strang, J., Griffiths, P., Taylor, C., Williamson, S., Fountain, J. and Gossop, M. (1999). Self-reported overdose among injecting drug users in London: extent and nature of the problem. *Addiction*, 94, pp. 471–78.

Rhodes, T. (1993). Time for community change: what has outreach to offer? *Addiction*, 68, pp. 1317–20.

Robertson, J. R., Bucknall, A., Welsby, P. O., Roberts, J. J. K., Inglis, J. M., Peutherer, J. F. and Brettle, R. P. (1986). Epidemic of AIDS-related virus (HTLV 3/LAV) infection among intravenous drug users. *British Medical Journal*, 292, pp. 527–29.

Russell, M. A. H., Wilson, C., Taylor, C. and Baker, C. D. (1979). Effect of general practitioners' advice against smoking. *British Medical Journal*, 21, pp. 231–35.

Sakol, M. S., Stark, C. and Sykes, R. (1989). Buprenorphine and temazepam abuse by drug takers in Glasgow: an increase. *British Journal of Addiction*, 1984, pp. 439–41.

Sheridan, J., Strang, J., Barber, N. and Glanz, A. (1996). Role of community pharmacies in relation to HIV prevention and drug misuse: findings from the 1995 national survey in England and Wales. *British Medical Journal*, 313, pp. 272–74.

Sheridan, J., Strang, J., Taylor, C. and Barber, N. (1997). HIV prevention and drug treatment services for drug misusers: a national study of community pharmacists' attitudes and their involvement in service specific training. *Addiction*, 92, pp. 1737–48.

Sheridan, J., Lovell, S., Turnbull, P., Parsons, J., Stimson, G. and Strang, J. (2000). Pharmacy-based needle exchange (PBNX) schemes in south east England: a survey of service providers. *Addiction*, 95, pp. 1551–60.

Simpson, D. D., Joe, G. W., Lehmann, W. E. K. and Sells, S. B. (1986). Addiction careers: aetiology, treatment and twelve-year follow-up outcomes. *Journal of Drug Issues*, 16, pp. 107–21.

Stimson, G. V. (1987). British drug clinics in the 1980s. *British Journal of Addiction*, 82, pp. 477–88.

Stimson, G. V. (1995). AIDS and injecting drug use in the United Kingdom, 1987–93: policy response and the prevention of the epidemic. *Social Science and Medicine*, 41, pp. 699–716.

Stimson, G. V. (1996). Has the UK averted an epidemic of HIV1 infection among drug injectors? *Addiction*, 91, pp. 1085–88.

Stimson, G. V. and Oppenheimer, E. (1982). *Heroin Addiction: treatment and control in Britain*. London: Tavistock.

Stimson, G. V., Alldritt, L., Dolan, K. and Donoghoe, M. (1988). Syringe exchange schemes for drug users in England and Scotland. *British Medical Journal*, 296, pp. 1717–19.

Stimson, G., Donoghoe, M., Lart, R. and Dolan, K. (1990). Distributing sterile needles and syringes to people who inject drugs: the syringe exchange experiment. In J. Strang and G. Stimson (eds), *AIDS and Drug Misuse* (pp. 222–31). London: Routledge.

Strain, E. C., Stitzer, M., Leibeson, I. A. *et al.* (1994). Comparison of buprenorphine and methadone in the treatment of opioid dependence. *American Journal of Psychiatry*, 151, pp. 1025–30.

Strang, J. (1984). Abstinence or abundance – what goal? *British Medical Journal*, 289, p. 604.

Strang, J. (1988). Changing injecting practices: blunting the needle habit (editorial). *British Journal of Addiction*, 83, pp. 237–39.

Strang, J. (1989). 'The British System': past, present and future. *International Review of Psychiatry*, 1, pp. 109–20.

Strang, J. (1990). Intermediate goals and the process of change. In J. Strang and G. Stimson (eds), *AIDS and Drug Misuse: the challenge for policy and practice in the 1990s* (pp. 211–21). London: Routledge.

Strang, J. (1992). Harm reduction for drug users: exploring the dimensions of harm, their measurement and strategies for their reduction. *AIDS and Public Policy Journal*, 7, pp. 145–52.

Strang, J. (1994). Drug misuse – the need to work with multiple indicators of change. In G. Edwards and M. Lader (eds), *Addiction: multiple processes of change* (pp. 217–30). Oxford: Oxford University Press.

Strang, J. and Gossop, M. (eds) (1994). *Heroin Addiction and Drug Policy: 'The British System'*. Oxford: Oxford University Press.

Strang, J. and Stimson, G. (eds) (1990). *AIDS and Drug Misuse: the challenge for policy and practice in the 1990s*. London and New York: Routledge.

Strang, J., Griffiths, P., Powis, B. and Gossop, M. (1992a). First use of heroin: changes in route of administration over time. *British Medical Journal*, 304, pp. 1222–23.

Strang, J., Des Jarlais, D. C., Griffiths, P. and Gossop, M. (1992b). The study of transitions in the route of drug use: the route from one route to another. *British Journal of Addiction*, 87, pp. 473–84.

Strang, J., Darke, S., Hall, W., Farrell, M. and Ali, R. (1996a). Heroin overdose: the case for take-home naloxone? *British Medical Journal*, 312, p. 1435.

Strang, J., Sheridan, J. and Barber, N. (1996b). Prescribing injectable and oral methadone to opiate addicts: results from the 1995 national survey of community pharmacies in England and Wales. *British Medical Journal*, 313, pp. 270–72.

Strang, J., Griffiths, P., Powis, B., Abbey, J. and Gossop, M. (1997a). How constant is an individual's route of heroin administration? Data from treatment and non-treatment samples. *Drug and Alcohol Dependence*, 46, pp. 115–18.

Strang, J., Finch, E., Hankinson, L., Farrell, M., Taylor, C. and Gossop, M. (1997b). Methadone treatment for opiate addiction: benefits in the first month. *Addiction Research*, 5, pp. 71–76.

Strang, J., Bacchus, L., Howes, S. and Watson, P. (1998). Turned away from treatment: maintenance-seeking opiate addicts at two-year follow-up. *Addiction Research*, 6, pp. 71–81.

Strang, J., Powis, B., Best, D., Vingoe, L., Griffiths, P., Taylor, C., Welch, S. and Gossop, M. (1999). Preventing opiate overdose fatalities with take-home naloxone: pre-launch study of possible impact and acceptability. *Addiction*, 94, pp. 199–204.

Strang, J. and Sheridan, J. (2003). Effect of national guidelines on prescription of methadone: analysis of NHS prescription data, England, 1990–2001. *British Medical Journal*, 327: 321–322.

Wallace, P., Cutler, S. and Haines, A. (1988). Randomised controlled trial of general practitioner intervention in patients with excessive alcohol consumption. *British Medical Journal*, 297, 663–68.

Ward, J., Mattick, R. and Hall, W. (1999). *Key Issues in Methadone Maintenance Treatment*. Sydney, Australia: University of New South Wales Press.

Winstock, A. R., Sheridan, J., Lovell, S., Farrell, M. and Strang, J. (2000). National survey of hepatitis testing and vaccination services provided by drug services in England and Wales. *European Journal of Clinical Microbiology and Infectious Diseases*, 19, pp. 823–28.

Chapter 17

Hepatitis C, the sleeping giant and the sleeping 'British System'

Tom Waller

Professor Miriam Alter from the United States first referred to the hepatitis C virus (HCV) as a sleeping giant in 1991 (Alter, 1991), both to emphasise the apparent size of HCV infection in the general population there and to highlight the fact that its most serious consequences were yet to be felt. Eight years later she was to demonstrate in a comprehensive general population survey that the prevalence in the USA general population was 1.8 per cent (Alter *et al.*, 1999). If we had an HCV epidemic of this size in Britain, a million people would be infected. It is clearly a very major new problem throughout the world – about 170 million people worldwide have been infected with hepatitis C. Yet in the UK there has to date been no accurate general population survey undertaken and no statistical projections for the future. We rely on mathematical estimates which, although valid in their own right, may considerably underestimate the size of the problem, leaving us unprepared to tackle the consequences of the epidemic.

Official calculations, based mainly on mathematical projections from HCV prevalence in antenatal clinics, suggest that approximately 0.5 per cent of the UK general population (about 300,000 people) have been infected with hepatitis C. This estimate is likely to be low, because since 1991 almost all new cases of HCV are believed to stem from injecting drug use and female drug users get pregnant at about half the rate of other women of the same age and residential profiles (Morrison *et al.*, 1995). In addition, significantly more injecting drug users are male (Johnson *et al.*, 1994), and men don't get pregnant. Nevertheless, if 300,000 of the UK general population are infected, this is numerically more than estimates for HIV. Clearly we have a major problem on our hands.

The mapping of HCV

In 1989 a specific test for HCV was discovered and over 95 per cent of all previous cases of Non-A, Non-B hepatitis (a diagnosis by exclusion) were shown to be hepatitis C. But even into the early 1990s, many doctors wrongly believed hepatitis C to be a mild disease of little clinical significance. In fact

80 per cent of those infected will develop chronic disease, many with progressive liver damage, and, if left untreated, in 30 years 30 per cent will die of liver cirrhosis, liver failure and primary liver cancer (Tong *et al.*, 1995; Poynard *et al.*, 1997).

Yet if so many people had been infected with hepatitis C, why were liver clinics not full of people dying from liver failure and liver cancer? The answer is that injecting drug use did not really take off in the UK until the late 1960s and the drug problem at that time was relatively small. Most people probably became infected with hepatitis C in the early and mid-1980s when shooting galleries were prevalent and one needle would circulate amongst dozens of people. To calculate the number at risk from infection by this route is not possible because it includes both past and present recreational and dependent injectors. Dependent stimulant injectors generally avoid drug services. Recreational drug use far exceeds dependent use. The 'at risk' population includes anyone who even injected once at a party. There are commonly no symptoms. Those who are symptomatic are usually overlooked because symptoms of tiredness and depression are non-specific. Most of those who contracted HCV are unaware of this but, unless they become aware that they may be infected and seek help, up to 90,000 people in the UK may die of HCV-induced disease by 2015 – more if the prevalence of HCV is higher than official statistics would suggest. A sudden and rapid rise in HCV disease and death can be anticipated in the UK. The United States is also forecasting a sudden increase in mortality from HCV disease.

The UK slowly wakes up to hepatitis C

How did the UK respond to the HCV epidemic when it first came to light? Understandably at first they concentrated on preventing HCV infection from blood transfusions, the injection of blood products and from organ transplants. Luckily viral inactivation had already been carried out on clotting factor treatment since 1985 (1987 in Scotland) to prevent HIV transmission to those with haemophilia and other clotting disorders. This would fortuitously also have prevented the transmission of HCV. In 1991 important steps were taken to prevent viral transmission from HCV-infected blood and blood products, and from organ transplants. All UK blood and organ donors have been screened for HCV since that time.

About 5,000 people were estimated to have been infected with HCV by blood transfusion prior to 1991, and figures from the UK Haemophilia Centre Directors' Organisation (to the end of 1999) state that 2,829 people with haemophilia or von Willibrand's (a related bleeding disorder) were exposed to untreated clotting factor concentrates before 1986. Yet this brings the total infected from these two important sources to less than 8,000 people. How did the very large number of infected people who remain contract HCV?

Evidence suggests that, unlike HIV, HCV is rarely transmitted sexually. About 5 per cent of HCV-positive mothers transmit the virus vertically to their children, and only a small proportion of infections appear to occur from sources other than injecting drug use (e.g. sharing toothbrushes and razors, tattooing, body-piercing, acupuncture, etc.). These sources only contribute towards a small part of the total UK pool of HCV infection, and from 1991 onwards almost all new infections are believed to have been via injecting drug use. What then was the government's response to HCV infection in drug users, and what was to be done about the very large numbers who had already been infected?

In fact, although anyone could have easily worked out that a blood-borne virus would be transmitted by shared injecting equipment, this was not picked up straight away. An examination of the literature on Non-A, Non-B hepatitis would have shown a high prevalence in injecting drug users from many places, but neither the drug field nor the government woke up to the enormity of this problem straight away. In 1991, an alert drug worker from West Suffolk, Roger Holmes, first noticed that many drug users were complaining of undue tiredness and malaise. Others had explained away such non-specific symptoms as the effects of lifestyle and street drug use, but Roger was not satisfied with this and in 1991 and 1992 he started testing drug users for hepatitis C. He found that of 142 HCV tests conducted on injecting drug users, 61 per cent were positive. If this was the finding in a remote corner of East Anglia what was happening elsewhere?

The first peer-reviewed British article on hepatitis C and drug use appeared in 1995 (Waller and Holmes, 1995). This article estimated from a retrospective study of recent HCV testing done by drug services throughout the UK that the average prevalence in injecting drug users was 60 per cent and that, extrapolating from the known prevalence in organ donors, the prevalence in the general population was probably about 400,000.

Drug policy inertia in the face of hepatitis C

Hepatitis C in drug users was first officially discussed in 1992 at the HIV working party of the Advisory Council on the Misuse of Drugs (ACMD) when the HIV and Drug Misuse Update report was being developed. In 1993 the subject was referred on to the full ACMD. The UK had been at the forefront of successful developments in national policy to prevent HIV transmission in injecting drug users; now was our chance to lead the world in developing a national strategy against an even bigger problem, the hepatitis C virus.

But this was not to be. The chairman of the ACMD decided to hand the matter over to the Department of Health. This had not happened with HIV, but it seemed reasonable at the time. ACMD members requested that an

ACMD working party should be set up to develop policy on HCV and drug users. There had after all been three ACMD reports on HIV. However, the Department of Health responded that they were unable to resource the administration of such a working party. This was a revelation to ACMD members. It was met with a stunned silence. Then an audible whisper with a strong Scottish accent could be heard, 'They doon't wanta knoow.' Clearly the brakes were being put on at a high level. The Department of Health did put on a day's discussion on HCV, but nothing came out of this, and the 'British System' shut its eyes to the problem.

Time passed. It seemed that at each meeting of the ACMD hepatitis C was raised and rejected. This led to increasing concern among a strong majority of members. The Department of Health's view remained that HCV was not a problem which required national action, and that they could not afford to resource an HCV working party. Rumours kept surfacing that the following words were reverberating around Richmond House (the Department of Health's headquarters), 'We had our fingers burnt with HIV and we are not going to do the same with hepatitis C.' What could be meant by this? British HIV policy had been amazingly successful and had saved the country much suffering and many hundreds of thousands of pounds.

At the ACMD, discussions on HCV with Department of Health attendants became increasingly acrimonious, but there was no movement. The ACMD's working party on drug-related deaths managed to include a chapter on HCV outlining its importance, but after six years of attempts to instigate progress through official channels there was no UK national strategy on hepatitis C or even one ACMD report.

The emergence of hepatitis C activism

Something needed to be done. In characteristic fashion Lorraine Hewitt, a longstanding ACMD member, said, 'What we need is a proper campaigning group to get things moving, and I'm going to set it up.' So it was that *Action on Hepatitis C* (AHC) was launched in July 1999. I was privileged to be its chair. There was already a small group in existence known as *C-Change*, which was the campaigning arm of the British Liver Trust, and had been funded by drug companies. But C-Change became worried that it might be counterproductive to highlight the fact that most people had become infected through injecting illicit drugs, and they focused on other modes of transmission.

AHC had no funding and its main primary aim was to achieve a national strategy on hepatitis C. If a good national strategy on hepatitis C was devised, properly funded and implemented, everything would flow from this. AHC members, all extremely busy in their own fields, gave up what little free time they had in order to obtain government action. Dr Graham Foster, a well-known hepatologist, and Dr Stephen Green, an infectious-disease consultant, were particularly active. Membership expanded to more than 50 and AHC became a formidable force of service users and professionals, hand-picked for their standing, influence in the field, and their desire to see progress. It included seven professors, and others well known in their various fields. Consultant representatives from hepatology, infectious disease and public health, epidemiologists, GPs, and professionals from the drug field, rubbed shoulders with service users who were actively engaged in improving services for drug users, such as Gary Sutton and Grant McNally. Several were past or present ACMD members. All had an equal say and the monthly meetings were attended by members from all over the UK.

The first nine months were spent meeting with officials from various departments, but this was resoundingly *un*successful. The Department of Health for England and Wales was adamant that there would be no national strategy developed for HCV. The ACMD minutes record that the chairman suggested the issue of hepatitis C should no longer be discussed. The only glimmer of light was from Scotland. Without any prompting from AHC, Scotland did begin to address the issues raised by the HCV epidemic with the publication of the *Scottish Needs Assessment Programme for Hepatitis C (SNAP)* (Office for Public Health, 2000) in March 2000 and *A Strategy for the Prevention and Management of Hepatitis C Infection in Greater Glasgow* (Greater Glasgow Health Board, 2000) in November 2000.

In May 2000, an extraordinary meeting of Action on Hepatitis C was held to discuss the failure to progress the issue. The outcome was a change of tack with approaches redirected to politicians and the media. Doors began to open almost immediately. In July 2000 AHC made a presentation to a joint meeting of the All Party Parliamentary Group on Drugs and the All Party Parliamentary Group on AIDS. Following this, several MPs and Lords asked parliamentary questions on hepatitis C. Some asked several questions: Lord Rea asked four in the House of Lords, Brian Iddon MP asked fifteen in the House of Commons.

At about this time drug users themselves were becoming increasingly angry about the lack of hepatitis C treatment availability in the UK and the lack of any national HCV strategy. Almost every other country in Europe now had a strategy or policy on HCV. Australia published its first HCV strategy in 1996 and was continuing to update it (Commonwealth Department of Health and Aged Care, 2000). National and local pressure groups started to emerge in the UK. Re-Act was the first national group starting in late 1999. The UK Assembly on Hepatitis C coordinated local groups and regional representatives. Mainliners, under the leadership of Basil Williams, was a driving force for many of these developments. It helped set up many groups, and hosted several influential international conferences on the virus. The UK Harm Reduction Alliance (UKHRA), chaired by Professor Gerry Stimson, was established in 2001 to help combat national drug policy moves away from individual and public health towards criminal justice issues.

A new national movement was taking place which included the setting up of other influential drug-user organisations such as the National Drug Users Development Agency and the Methadone Alliance.

The new mobilised response – but still reticent

Against this background of increasing political and public pressure things suddenly started to happen. In October 2000 NICE officially approved the use of combined interferon/ribavirin treatment for HCV in the UK (National Institute for Clinical Excellence, 2000). The following month, with the help of parliamentary lobbying from C-Change, there was a debate on hepatitis C in the House of Lords. Then the Department of Health rapidly formulated guidelines on hepatitis C for professionals who were working with drug users. These were published in March 2001. The same month a national HCV Strategy Working Group for England and Wales was officially established with a remit to report in one year. In April 2001 a group was established to define a strategy for HCV in London. In November 2001 there was a 90-minute House of Commons adjournment debate on hepatitis C, organised and led by Brian Iddon MP, and various newspaper articles and TV documentaries on hepatitis C started to appear. By the end of the year an HCV strategic working party was established for Northern Ireland. Within the space of just over twelve months, there had been a complete about-turn in national policy and many new initiatives.

Much change is required to prevent the spread of the virus and to reduce secondary damage to those who are already infected with the virus. Needle exchange, which had been set up in the late 1980s to contain the spread of HIV, had been shown fortuitously to also help prevent HCV transmission. To contain the spread of HCV a doubling in the uptake of needle exchange facilities is needed, together with changes in advice and legislation to prevent HCV spread via injecting paraphernalia. More outreach services are required and drug treatment services need to change to attract stimulant injectors. Opiate injectors must have faster access to oral methadone. The problem of drug treatment services failing to address alcohol use must be countered. Alcohol escalates HCV disease progression. Although some good epidemiological research has already been done on HCV in drug users, particularly by the Centre for Research on Drugs and Health Behaviour, considerably more money needs to be spent on research. We don't even know basic things such as how to most effectively kill the virus following a blood spill and we need good general population studies.

With regard to HCV treatment, huge numbers in the UK are about to pass the point of no return when liver failure will appear, treatable only by liver transplants. Even using split livers, transplants are becoming dangerously close to running out. France had a national target to reach 85 per cent of their HCV-infected population by 2003. There needs to be a massive national publicity campaign throughout the UK to make people aware of the various at-risk groups, particularly injecting drug users, and to ask them to come forward for confidential HCV testing if they think they have been at risk. The treatment system must be robust enough to cope with the numbers of people who come forward. More specialist HCV services are required. Accurate projections of the epidemic in future years are needed now to ensure that enough doctors and nurses are properly trained.

How effective have the early initiatives been? One year after the NICE first report on HCV drug treatment had been published, the British Liver Trust found that more money had been spent on liver transplants in the UK than on drug treatment for hepatitis C. The NICE recommendations had made no difference. Before the NICE report in October 2000 there had been postcode prescribing (Rosenberg, 2001) and it continued afterwards (Foster and Chapman, 2000). In many parts of the country there is still no treatment available or it is strictly limited. In some places HCV testing has been prevented.

Undoubtedly the reticence to grapple with the HCV problem has been fuelled by the high costs of treatment and the repeated rejection of centralised funding by government. The cost of the drugs for one person's treatment is about £8,000. Taking into account investigations, which may include a liver biopsy, and other costs, figures charged by different NHS Trusts vary from £12,000 to £15,000. Improved drug treatment for HCV, using pegylated interferon, is usually life-saving and easier to comply with, but is more expensive. Given the numbers involved it is easy to see why some officials hope drug users can be left to die without much public reaction.

In the United States, where 2.7 million people are infected with HCV, the total cost of the HCV epidemic in 1997 was estimated to be 5.46 billion dollars (Leigh et al., 2001). This is comparable to the national costs of asthma and rheumatoid arthritis, but neither of those two diseases is forecast to increase their burden as rapidly as hepatitis C. In spite of the cost, treatment has been shown to save money and America is treating as many people as possible.

Discrimination against drug users

One difficulty, not completely confined to the UK, is that many professional guidelines have unjustly excluded drug injectors from HCV treatment. The European Association for the Study of the Liver (EASL) consensus statement (International Consensus Conference on Hepatitis C, 1999), the NICE guidelines on combined interferon–ribavirin treatment of HCV (National Institute for Clinical Excellence, 2000), and clinical guidelines on the management of hepatitis C by the British Society of Gastroenterology (British Society of Gastroenterology, 2001) have excluded 'in general' all current injecting drug users from treatment. The NICE guidelines do allow exceptions but these are open to interpretation. The onus is on the drug user to reliably assure the prescribing clinician that re-infection, compliance and drug interactions pose no problems. When discrimination against injecting drug users is known to be rife, and with extreme pressure to cut back on health spending, this reliance on interpretation is a major concern. A denial of treatment of HCV to anyone when the illness is life-threatening is a serious matter and infringes human rights. These guidelines and the lack of centralised funding for HCV treatment have undoubtedly led to greatly increased morbidity and mortality of drug users, making inconsequential moves by the Department of Health to reduce drug-related deaths.

Two scientific papers of particular importance were published in the medical press in 2001. The first by seven authors from the University of California in San Francisco (UCSF) (Edlin *et al.*, 2001) reflects the consensus of a group of 38 national and international experts on AIDS, liver disease, substance abuse and health policy. It lays out the evidence why injecting and other drug users should not be denied treatment for HCV. The second from a German group (Backmund *et al.*, 2001) showed that current injectors not only can be treated successfully for HCV, but show greater compliance than other patients. It is hoped that subsequent guidelines, NICE recommendations, and the new UK HCV strategies will take these papers into account.

Any HCV strategy must address the thorny problem of hepatitis C and prisons. UK prisons generate much HCV. A lack of availability of sterile injecting equipment puts pressure on drug-using prisoners to share. Some countries have developed successful prison needle exchanges. Elsewhere unsterile tattooing has been shown to be a major source of blood-borne virus transmission among prisoners (Holsen *et al.*, 1993). To date these findings have been relatively ignored in the UK. Other difficulties include the exemption of most UK prisoners from accessing treatment for HCV – a problem compounded by the movement of prisoners.

Conclusion

None of the problems surrounding HCV are insurmountable if the will and funds are there. But let us be clear about the major tasks immediately in front of us. Clearly defined and comprehensive UK HCV strategies must now emerge; they must be properly funded and implemented; and better guidelines for the treatment of drug users with HCV still need to be developed.

References

A Strategy for the Prevention and Management of Hepatitis C Infection in Greater Glasgow (2000) Greater Glasgow Health Board: Glasgow.

Alter, M. J. (1991) Hepatitis C: a sleeping giant? *American Journal of Medicine*, 91 (3B), pp. 112S–115S.

Alter, M. J., Kruszon-Moran, D., Nainan, O. V. *et al.* (1999) The prevalence of hepatitis C virus infection in the United States, 1988 through to 1994. *New England Journal of Medicine*, 341, pp. 556–562.

Backmund, M., Meyer, K., Von Zielonka, M. and Eichenlaub, D. (2001) Treatment of hepatitis C infection in injecting drug users. *Hepatology*, 34 (1), pp. 188–193.

British Society of Gastroenterology (BSG) (2001) *Clinical Guidelines on the management of hepatitis C*. http://www.bsg.org.uk/guidelines/clinguidehepc.html

EASL International Consensus Conference on Hepatitis C. Consensus Statement. (1999) *Journal of Hepatology*, 30, pp. 956–961.

Edlin, B. R., Seal, K. H., Lorvick, J. *et al.* (2001) Is it justifiable to withhold treatment for hepatitis C from illicit drug users? *New England Journal of Medicine*, 345 (3), pp. 211–214.

Foster, G. R. and Chapman, R. (2000) Combination treatment for hepatitis C is not being given. *British Medical Journal*, 321, p. 899.

Holsen, D., Harthug, S. and Myrmel, H. (1993) Prevalence of antibodies to hepatitis C virus and association with intravenous drug abuse and tattooing in a national prison in Norway. *European Journal of Clinical Microbiology and Infectious Diseases*, 12, pp. 673–676.

Johnson, A. M., Wadsworth, J., Wellings, K. and Field, J. (1994) *Sexual Attitudes and Lifestyles*. London: Blackwell Scientific Publications, pp. 271–273.

Leigh, J., Bowlus, C. L., Leistikow, B. N. and Schenker, M. (2001) Costs of hepatitis C. *Archives of Internal Medicine*, 161, pp. 2231–2237.

Morrison, C. L., Ruben, S. M. and Beeching, N. J. (1995) Female sexual health problems in a drug dependency unit. *International Journal of STD and AIDS*, 6, pp. 201–203.

National Hepatitis C Strategy 1999–2000 to 2003–2004 (2000) Commonwealth of Australia: Commonwealth Department of Health and Aged Care.

National Institute for Clinical Excellence (NICE) (2000) *Guidance on the Use of Ribavirin and Interferon Alpha for Hepatitis C*. www.nice.org.uk

Office for Public Health in Scotland (2000) *Scottish Needs Assessment Programme (SNAP), Hepatitis C*, Glasgow.

Poynard, T., Bedossa, P. and Opolon, P. (1997) for the OBSVIRC, CLINIVIR and DOSVIRC groups. Natural history of liver fibrosis progression in patients with chronic hepatitis C. *Lancet*, 349, pp. 825–832.

Rosenberg, D., (2001) Personal communication of a postal survey. Letter to Dr G. Foster.

Tong, M., El-Farrah, N., Reikes, A. and Co, R. (1995) Clinical outcomes after transfusion associated hepatitis C virus. *New England Journal of Medicine*, 332, pp. 1463–1466.

Waller, T. and Holmes, R. (1993) Hepatitis C: time to wake up. *Druglink*, 8 (3), pp. 7–9.

Waller, T. and Holmes, R. (1995) Hepatitis C: scale and impact in Britain. *Druglink*, 10 (5), pp. 8–11.

Index

Note: page numbers in Volume 1 in normal type, in Volume 2 in bold. Figures and tables in italics